'Without the presence and acceptance of
the midwife, obstetrics becomes aggressive,
technological and inhuman.' –

Professor G.J. Kloosterman,
*formerly of the Department of Obstetrics and Gynaecology,
University of Amsterdam Hospital, the Netherlands*

CONTENTS

DEFINITION OF A MIDWIFE

'A person who, having been regularly admitted to a midwifery educational program duly recognized in the jurisdiction in which it is located, has successfully completed the prescribed course of studies in midwifery and has acquired the requisite qualifications to be registered and/or legally licensed to practice midwifery.

The sphere of practice: she must be able to give the necessary supervision, care and advice to women during pregnancy, labor and postpartum period, to conduct deliveries on her own responsibility, and to care for the newborn and the infant. This care includes preventive measures, the detection of abnormal conditions in mother and child, the procurement of medical assistance, and the execution of emergency measures in the absence of medical help.

She has an important task in counseling and education – not only for patients, but also within the family and community. The work should involve antenatal education and preparation for parenthood and extends to certain areas of gynecology, family planning and child care.

She may practice in hospitals, clinics, health units, domiciliary conditions or any other service.' (World Health Organisation, 1966)

WHY WOMEN NEED MIDWIVES

SHEILA KITZINGER

In childbirth today the obstetrician usually stands centre-stage. The midwife is invisible. Yet historically, ever since the first recorded accounts of birth, and in countries all over the world, midwives have had the main responsibility for giving care before, during and after a baby is born, and in many societies today the health of most mothers and newborn babies still depends on midwives. Midwives are the experts in normal childbirth, and in giving care which prevents the development of the abnormal.

The midwife shares the experience with the woman giving birth. She is literally 'mid' or 'with' her in an empathic, intimate relationship ('midwife' comes from the Anglo-Saxon literally meaning 'with woman'), while the obstetrician 'stands in front of' the woman. The midwife is also the wise woman, the *'sage femme'* who understands women's rhythms and the mysteries of birth and death. Two thousand five hundred years ago, the Tao Te Ching described the role of the midwife thus:

> You are a midwife: you are assisting at someone else's birth. Do good without show or fuss. Facilitate what is happening rather than what you think ought to be happening. If you must take the lead, lead so that the mother is helped, yet still free and in charge. When the baby is born, the mother will rightly say: 'We did it ourselves!'[1]

Though there have been histories of midwifery and midwifery texts, there has never been a book which explores what it means to be a midwife in different social and medical systems and the problems which midwifery faces in the world today. Midwives themselves often do not know how those in other countries work or what their main concerns are. They may not realise that the changes taking place in childbirth, the new articulation of needs and wishes by women having babies, and the banding together and campaigning of midwives and mothers to improve the birth experience, is occurring in many different parts of the world. It is an international movement which started because of women's dissatisfaction with the obstetric system and with factory-farm conditions in childbirth, a movement which now in the late 1980s is gathering momentum and power.

In some countries midwives are isolated, and it is difficult for them to see their midwifery in a wider social context. Perhaps it is not surprising that South African midwives, whether Black, Coloured or White, have little opportunity of knowing what is happening in the rest of the world. But there are also many midwives in Europe who are equally unaware that they are part of a world movement in which midwives thousands of miles apart share the same concerns and are trying to work out their relations with doctors and with the women in their care. They do not realise that midwives everywhere are not just reacting to change, but are creating change, evolving a new art of midwifery while at the same time rediscovering the ancient art.

When midwives seek change merely at a personal level, or in the setting of one hospital, they usually end up feeling frustrated. It is essential for them to gain a broad view and act in awareness of the world-wide sisterhood of midwives. Only thus can they be politically effective and redress the balance of power between obstetricians and midwives, which at present is heavily weighted towards obstetrics. It is a top-heavy medical hierarchy in which midwives are treated, on the whole, as assistants to doctors and low-status members of a system over which they have no control.

MIDWIFERY IN THE PAST

The history of midwifery has been a long struggle between, firstly, a male-dominated priesthood and, subsequently, a system of organised medicine also controlled by men, and a women's community-based network of helping and healing.[2] Healing was initially an extension of mothering and every woman was expected to have some medical and nursing skills. There were powerful religious elements in birth and midwives drew on these, as well as using their practical skills, for safe delivery. The great goddesses of creation were also those of healing and of birth.

Some of the earliest references to midwives occur in the ancient Egyptian *Ebers Papyrus*, one of the first midwifery textbooks. In Egypt surgery was usually done by the priest. Normal childbirth was the task of the midwives. In the Old Testament we are told that Jewish midwives defied Egyptian rulers:

> The King of Egypt spake to the Hebrew Midwives . . . 'When ye do the office of a midwife to the Hebrew women, and see them upon the stools [low birth stools shaped like horseshoes which allowed the labouring women to be in a supported modified squatting posture for birth] . . . if it be a son, then ye shall kill him; but if it be a daughter then she shall live.' But the midwives feared God, and did not as the King of Egypt commanded them but saved the men children alive. And the King of Egypt called for the midwives and said unto them, 'Why have you done this thing, and have saved the children alive?' And the midwives said unto Pharaoh, 'Because the Hebrew women are not as the Egyptian women; for they are lively, and are delivered ere the midwives come in unto them.'

Women were excluded from medical schools in ancient Greece and most women healers became midwives, though some midwives wrote books on abortion and infertility. Because midwifery was a woman's job it had low status. One Athenian midwife disguised herself as a man, perhaps because only then was she able to perform Caesarean sections.

Women were excluded from medical schools in Rome, too. By the third century BC women in medicine, and in particular midwives, were ridiculed by male writers as superstitious peasants, drunks, sorcerers and poisoners. Though wealthy people had private hospitals, the poor sought help from 'wise women' and midwives, some of whom were the earliest Christian martyrs.

In later Christianity, healing was vested in the priesthood. Throughout the Dark Ages many midwives were burned as witches, for though the church tolerated women healers if they were subservient to ecclesiastic rules, it was hostile to any woman who dared to practise independently. These women represented a challenge to the authority of the church and risked being burned as witches. This kind of female healing was seen as a pagan, evil practice, derived from the Devil. The *Malleus Maleficarium* denounced midwives because they 'surpass all other witches in their crimes'. A law was passed in 1512 that all midwives had to be licensed by the Bishop's Court. In 1584 it was decreed that midwives had to take an oath not to use 'any witchcraft, charms, relics, or invocation to any saint in the time of Travail'.

The witch-hunt ended first in the Netherlands, and midwives from many other European countries travelled to Holland to get certificates in midwifery, which would stand them in good stead if they were later accused of witchcraft.

By the second decade of the seventeenth century male surgeons were already supplanting midwives at births in the noble families of France, and the term 'man midwife' had been introduced into English. Over the next hundred years, throughout Europe, male apothecaries and surgeons did more and more midwifery. The professionalisation of healing had started in Europe during the Middle Ages when the first colleges and guilds were formed. Everywhere except in Italy women were excluded from universities and so could not get formal training or qualifications.

> The status of an occupation depends not only on the financial rewards received by its leading members, but also on their ability to distinguish themselves from the untrained 'irregular' practitioners of their art and from those whose morals offend against the ruling code of behaviour.[3]

Medical men joined corporate bodies such as the College of Physicians and the Company of Surgeons, but midwives were usually poor and ill-educated, and even when they had wealth and education were not organised to gain formal recognition or professional status.

The medical men denounced midwives as 'cackling dames' who prescribed 'kitchen physics'. The use of instruments was restricted to male *accoucheurs*, and even they were in hot competition with one another. After Peter Chamberlen invented the forceps, they were kept a closely guarded secret between the Chamberlens for one hundred years.

From the seventeenth century on midwives have been expected to concede to doctors, and, however highly experienced they are, to listen to the advice and obey the instructions of men who were often 'without practical experience, and sometimes little relevant theoretical knowledge, but who had greater prestige by virtue of their profession and gender'.[4]

Yet most medicine and surgery remained basically domestic arts. A housekeeping book of 1700 says that women should 'have competent knowledge of Physick and Chyrugery that they may be able to help their maimed, sick and indigent Neighbours for Commonly all good and Charitable Ladies make this a part of their housekeeping business'.[5] If a doctor was called in, he worked under the critical eye of women of the household and had to explain, justify and defend every action he took. Except in dire emergency, he could not simply come in and take over.

In the nineteenth century the rising middle classes came to prefer obstetric care to the traditional care from midwives. Right through the century, however, the poor had recourse to midwives because doctors were not interested in doing midwifery among the working class. They resisted attempts to organise midwifery and make it a profession in case it affected their lucrative middle class practices.

Victorian midwives charged about a quarter of the average doctor's fee. They stayed in the home for at least nine days after delivery to look after mother and baby and often did the household cooking, cleaning and laundry, as peasant midwives continue to do in many countries today. They were often literally 'old wives' who had large families of their own and handed down what they had learned from practical experience. Women sought their help on all aspects of fertility and infertility.

The great mother goddesses of Anatolia, Egypt and Greece, represented as birth-giving and providing power and skill to the midwife, had been overtaken by a stern father God. And by the nineteenth century midwives themselves, formerly attributed with special spiritual insights and religious qualities, had often been degraded to backstreet abortionists.[6]

In 1824 the British Lying-in Hospital in London began to train 'monthly nurses', because male doctors wanted to have a woman around who would save them having to be present throughout labour, and to take care of the mess and look after the mother afterwards. By 1844 there were three times as many of these nurses in training as midwives.[7] The midwives' professional and social status had fallen to rock bottom.

Though doctors were doing more and more deliveries, birth did not become safer. In the first half of the twentieth century many women still did not survive it. Almost as many died in 1903 as had fifty years earlier; in England the maternal mortality rate in 1847 was 6 per 1,000; in 1903 it was 4 per 1,000.[8] In fact, the rate did not drop below 1 per 1,000 until 1944. Death rates of those women who were delivered at home by midwives were much lower than those delivered in the maternity hospitals and workhouses, where 'unnecessary intervention in normal labours on a huge scale was accompanied by inadequate antisepsis'. Newly delivered mothers were at risk of contracting puerperal fever when doctors attended women in childbirth with unwashed hands after having come from examining sick patients or doing an autopsy. In home birth with a midwife there was less chance of cross-infection and puerperal fever, the main cause of maternal death at that time.[9]

In the United States maternal mortality 'remained more or less constant at one of the largest recorded levels in the world although a large and rapidly growing proportion of deliveries after 1920 took place in hospital under the care of specialist obstetricians.'

The Midwives' Act passed by the British Parliament in 1902 arose out of concern to build a professional basis for midwifery. It laid down that no woman could use the title of midwife unless registered with the Central Midwives Board, and this set the scene for the coming of the modern midwife.

Yet the historical struggle between midwives and the male-dominated medical Establishment has persisted in all countries of the world throughout the twentieth century.

THE SPECIAL QUALITIES OF THE MIDWIFE

Being a midwife, as distinct from being an assistant to the obstetrician and someone who merely carries out his orders, strikes at the very basis of male power in medicine.

To a large extent the modern safety of birth has come about because of improved social conditions, which have resulted in better health among childbearing women. Contraception, termination of pregnancy and women's new-found ability to control, at least in part, if and when to have babies, have also contributed to safer birth. When improved social conditions increase the likelihood of straightforward physiological, rather than surgical, childbirth, the logical conclusion might be that obstetricians are made largely redundant. Women then need midwives, the guardians of normal childbirth, rarely obstetricians. It is understandable, therefore, that, having no obvious function, doctors become anxious about their role and intervene in perfectly normal labours. They do this also because the technology is there, waiting to be used, because they have been trained to intervene and believe their skills are necessary, and because they suffer from what is to midwives a well-known anxiety state – seeing themselves as saviours and defenders of the foetus, the only ones who really *care* – which leads to intrusive and sometimes iatrogenic (disease-producing) intervention. It is not foetal distress that is the cause of the trouble, but obstetricians' distress.

Midwives today are not quite sure *who* they are or what they want to be. And maternity care systems often seem even less certain about the role and function of midwives. There are three stereotypes of the midwife. She can be the vicious old meddler and witch, one fingernail long and sharpened ready to puncture the membranes, to perform an episiotomy, or to pierce the baby's fontanelle. A nineteenth-century example of this is Sarah Gamp in Dickens's *Martin Chuzzlewit*, who reels drunkenly from laying out the dead to catching babies. The second is the romantic image of the warm, wise woman who instinctively understands other women's needs, who dedicates herself to them with complete selflessness, and who is always ready with less healing herbs and her embracing, comforting arms. Then there is the cool, professional expert who sits in front of a bank of remote control electronic foetal monitors making management decisions, all the processes of labour under micro-chip control. None of these stereotypes reflects the reality of midwifery.

The contrast between the stereotypes of the romantic and the super professional image implies a dichotomy between caring on the one hand and expertise on the other, as if midwives can only be caring if they are purely intuitive and can only exercise the intellect when using expensive and complicated machines to intervene in a natural physiological process. This polarity is typical of much thinking in obstetrics, as if the caregiver must choose between the old 'bedside manner', with its connotations of the bearded nineteenth-century doctor watching over the patient dying of pneumonia, and, in contrast, the surgeon-saviour, intellectually vigorous, emotionally detached, powerful to control women's wayward bodies. Every TV film about a 'woman's problem' ends with the authorised gynaecological judgment delivered by one such expert, in which our own knowledge about our bodies, our own feelings, are dismissed as trivial, subjective, anecdotal – even hysterical.

The polarisation of images of the midwife is not just inaccurate. It is dangerously wrong. For the midwife cannot be skilled without being caring. She cannot be truly caring without being skilled. All those who work with childbearing women owe it to them to develop skills and knowledge, and to question all received opinion, including that in the obstetric and midwifery textbooks, to take nothing for granted just because we want to believe it. It is also the responsibility of every one of us to examine critically *all* dogmas, including those enshrined in scientific terminology, to ask for the evidence and investigate the benefits and hazards of such things as shaving of the perineum, enemas and suppositories, putting women to bed in labour, routine intravenous infusions, commanded pushing and pro-longed breath-holding in the second stage, routine episiotomy, and every one of the rules and regulations and customary practices current in hospitals today.

The obstetrician's role is distinct from that of the midwife in that he (and, apart from the Soviet Union, in most countries the majority of obstetricians are male) defines childbirth in exclusively medical terms. A woman having a baby wants to feel secure in the knowledge that her health and that of her baby is assured. But this is not all. For her the coming of this child has other meanings in her personal life and relationships. The midwife is as concerned as the obstetrician with the physical aspects of birth, but she also needs to be aware of emotional changes and the social context of birth. This demands a great deal of confidence, sound basic knowledge and clinical experience. She focuses on women's experiences, not only on medical events. She knows how to watch and wait, how to bide her time when this is the right thing to do, how to surrender management and, while still alert and observant, nurture the natural process. An American midwife expresses it in this way: 'The essence of midwifery is staying sensitively in the moment – in other words, being humble and paying attention. But this simple focus can easily be destroyed by the desire for control. . . . The wise midwife . . . understands ebb and flow.'[10]

EMPIRICAL MIDWIVES

In Third World countries up to three-quarters of all births are attended by women whom the World Health Organisation (WHO) calls 'traditional birth attendants'. Sometimes these are simply women who have had children themselves and who are around when a baby is born – often the husband's mother and sisters or a woman's own kin.

In many traditional cultures, however, among the group of women who support a woman in childbirth there is one who has learned special midwifery skills and who orchestrates what happens in the birthing room. She is the empirical or 'lay' midwife. In Jamaica, for example, she is known as the *nana*, in Malaysia as the *bidankampung*. She belongs to the local community, speaks the same language and dialect, already knows the woman and her family well, shares the same system of beliefs about health and illness, is readily available, and is either paid in kind or charges very little. She is usually expert in a variety of comfort techniques and ways of assisting the birth by transforming the woman's psychological state.

As western-style medical systems have been introduced in developing countries, empirical midwives have usually been downgraded, and often outlawed. Instead of working through them to achieve greater safety, an alien system has been introduced which is often completely unsuitable for local conditions, and to which the majority of women have no access. WHO believes that 'traditional birth attendants constitute an important resource that could be mobilised to help achieve the social goal of health for all'.[11]

The development of midwifery services is vital for the health of women and families in the Third World, and trained midwives will have an important task to play in reaching out to, learning from, and working alongside traditional empirical midwives, and helping them make their practice as effective, caring and safe as possible.

MISUSE OF MIDWIVES

In the modern health care system the midwife has often disappeared altogether, as she has in North America. When she does exist, she is used as a nurse rather than as a midwife. She does not possess the privilege or status of the doctor and is expected to work under his instructions. Even in those countries where most babies are delivered by midwives, the midwife's role has been fragmented. Her work has become task-centred rather than woman-centred, so that she cannot build a relationship with the mother, and she is denied much of the vocational satisfaction which led her to midwifery in the first place. She is unable to use her special skills, and may also lose her sensitivity.

When there is no continuity of care midwives tend to be used interchangeably with nurses – as agents of crowd control in the antenatal clinic, and frequently only to perform routine tasks such as weighing, taking blood pressure and testing urine. As a result, a midwife may meet the woman having a baby for the first time when she is in labour. Under these circumstances midwives feel they are working on an assembly line and it is difficult or impossible for them to know and understand the needs of women in their care.[12]

In the women's movement and the childbirth movement – and until the 1980s these have been very separate – the role of the midwife has been extolled as representing sisterhood, in contrast to the authoritarianism and paternalism of the obstetrician. As a result, in many countries women have in the 1980s developed a very positive image of midwives. It comes as a shock when they find that midwives, too, can be authoritarian. Yet midwives themselves can become institutionalised, trapped in the medical system and under constant pressure from it, and may forget their unique role. They then use their energy in supporting and maintaining the existing institutional structure, are frightened of change, readily feel under attack when policies are questioned, may try to reinforce their own status by treating women like naughty and irresponsible children, and are concerned to please those further up the hospital hierarchy, who are their judges, and on whom their jobs depend, rather than giving priority to their relationships with the women in their care.

Studies of relations between midwives and women carried out by midwives themselves reveal that the hospital system often makes it difficult for midwives to build positive, cooperative relationships, and that they may use a variety of strategies, albeit unconsciously, to block discussion, resist giving information, restrict choice and insulate themselves from those in their care.[13] Even when they do talk with pregnant women they frequently only describe procedures, and avoid discussing the advantages and disadvantages of different practices. Some midwives regularly put obstacles in the way of discussion developing; it may be that they do not know how to encourage it or that they dislike any kind of mutual dialogue. Junior midwives may feel it is wise to say as little as possible, perhaps because they do not always know the answers themselves. Yet women tend to ask more questions of junior staff because they are usually with them longer.

Some midwives are so concerned to keep routines flowing smoothly that this is given higher priority than talking with women. They may be so rushed that when they do give information women often cannot understand it because it is presented in such large packages. On the whole, though, reassurance is provided in the place of information. When a midwife realises that a woman is worrying about something, she may tell her, in effect, that there is no reason for her anxiety, and so devalues her emotions:

Patient: 'I'm scared.'
Midwife: 'You mustn't be scared.'
(Silence, delivered eight minutes later.)[14]

Finally, some midwives are happier working with machines than with women. When the machines go wrong there may be more 'conversation' with them than with women in labour.

In seeking greater recognition of the importance of midwives we should not assume that it is merely a matter of changing professional and public perceptions of midwifery. Much must also be done to explore midwives' own awareness of what they can give, to increase their sensitivity to the needs of women and families, and to create new standards of care and caring in which midwives 'see women as allies in a wider search for knowledge and change'.[15] In many countries this is happening, sparked by the 'ginger' movements which have involved women and midwives working together in pressure groups to improve maternity care. But to romanticise midwifery is to do a disservice to the profession, by failing to recognise the work that needs to be done by midwives themselves to explore their role and to fully realise their capacity to be 'with' women in childbirth and experience the deep satisfaction that this brings.

Nowadays most women have to give birth surrounded by strangers in an alien and often frightening environment. This means that the midwife has to overcome tremendous obstacles in trying to make personal contact and to work *with* the woman in labour instead of merely *on* her. There is an acute shortage of midwives in many countries, and those remaining work in understaffed units and are overworked and exploited by a medical system which they feel powerless to change.

Midwives are not only in subordinate relation to doctors. They are also subject to hospital administration. The immediate goals of administrators concern finance and maintenance, the control of staff and the prestige of the institution. Under economic pressure, their primary aim is financial stability, economy and functional efficiency. There may be only a tenuous link between these goals and the quality of care given to women.

Because midwives are deeply concerned about what is happening to women and their babies, they often lose satisfaction in their jobs and leave. In Britain only one in five qualified midwives is actually practising, and most women who start to do midwifery leave within five years. Others stay as midwives, but give up the struggle and treat women having babies like any other product on a conveyor belt passing in front of them.

This process began when childbirth was moved from home to hospital. No longer a friend in the house and regular guest during pregnancy, the midwife became part of a team. As such, she was, and remains, under pressure to give her primary allegiance to that team rather than to the woman giving birth.

The introduction of childbirth technology has intensified this process of change. It means that some aspects of the management of labour have been taken over entirely by doctors. Depending on the country and the particular hospital, ultrasound visaging may have replaced the midwife's laying on of hands and abdominal palpation, and midwives may not be relied on to monitor the foetal heart with a Pinard's stethoscope (the traditional trumpet stethoscope) or be permitted to perform a vacuum extraction. The technological revolution has also meant that in many countries midwives are expected to develop skills in handling electronic machinery and in recording and interpreting data. While we may welcome this acknowledgment of the midwife's competence, her new task of dealing with electronics can detract from her relationship with the woman for whom she is caring and have the effect of eroding clinical skills – those of observation, watchful expectancy and hands-on midwifery. It leads inevitably to an undervaluing of her experience, the knowledge that comes from human contact and her insight into the way a woman's body is working and the pattern of her labour, and her awareness of how she feels and what is on her mind. In concentrating exclusively on the action of the uterus, it is easy to forget that this organ is part of a woman, and that the most effective way of encouraging uterine efficiency may be the one-to-one care of a good midwife and the strong emotional support that she can give.

THE DANGER OF DOMINATION BY OBSTETRICS

It might be expected that those societies that have most doctors have the most highly evolved maternity care. But it is those care systems which value midwives, and in which midwives have greatest responsibility in birth – the Scandinavian countries and the Netherlands – which have the lowest perinatal mortality rates. In Italy, for example, midwives have very low status. Deliveries are conducted by obstetricians, and there is an excess of doctors all competing for custom. In 1984, the latest year for which we have directly comparable figures, the Italian perinatal mortality rate was 14.5 per 1,000 compared with 10 in the Netherlands, 8.4 in Denmark, 7.6 in Finland and 7.3 in Sweden – all countries where midwifery is strong. In 1981, at the time of writing the latest date for which United States figures were published, the perinatal mortality rate was 13.4 in the country where midwifery was almost completely destroyed by the medical system.[16]

In terms of perinatal outcome midwife care compares very favourably with that from obstetricians.[17] In Britain a study that compared GP unit care with consultant care in one hospital actually focused on care given by community midwives, in contrast to that coming from obstetric teams in which the consultant was the senior member of a hierarchy where midwives were the lowest paid and most junior members. The women in this study were all classified as low-risk and were allocated to community midwife or consultant unit care depending on where they lived in the area. When they had personal care from community midwives women had fewer inductions, went into hospital in a more advanced state of labour, received less pethidine and fewer epidurals, had less electronic field monitoring, less augmentation of labour with oxytocin and fewer forceps deliveries, and foetal distress was not diagnosed so often and babies were not intubated so frequently. The one minute Apgar score was under 6 (indicating that the newborn was short of oxygen) in only 1.6 per cent of babies cared for by the community midwives compared with 17.5 per cent of those in the consultant team system of care.[18]

A pilot project using certified nurse-midwives was set up in California in the 1960s in Madera County, and special legislation was passed making midwifery lawful while the project lasted. In the first eighteen months of the project the prematurity rate dropped from 11 per cent to 6.6 per cent and the neonatal mortality rate from 23.9 per 1,000 to 10.3 per 1,000. In spite of these positive results, the California Medical Society continued to oppose the permanent legislation of nurse-midwifery and the project ceased. After the nurse-midwives had left, the prematurity rate increased by almost 50 per cent and the neonatal mortality rate tripled.[19] In all countries where there is a choice between obstetrician and midwife care – which in practice works out as obstetricians for the better-off and midwives for the poorest women – those who can pay for a private obstetrician have much higher rates of intervention in childbirth, including Caesarean section. In parts of Latin America, for example, well over 50 per cent of upper-class women are delivered by Caesarean section, whereas nearly 90 per cent of peasant women give birth vaginally. Yet it might be supposed that women with good nutrition, and who live in comfort, would be healthier and have less need of intervention than undernourished and impoverished women. There seems to be something about the kind of care midwives offer that enhances a woman's ability to give birth without intervention, and avoids the pathological situations in which intervention is deemed necessary.

In many traditional cultures, especially in Third World societies, birth is seen as an act in which a woman draws on her own inner power, and if there are difficulties these are perceived as posing dilemmas in terms of the spiritual life and relationships between those involved in the birth of that child, rather than as presenting technical and mechanical problems. The midwife is mediator of these difficult relationships, a guide on the journey in which a woman confronts these spiritual and psychological challenges.

In contemporary western thinking (and to a large extent throughout the history of the western world) there is a dislocation between mind and body, an antithesis between the spiritual and the physical. The history of obstetrics is a record of men's struggle to construct a system of scientific certainties on which the management of labour can be based, and to eliminate women's inconvenient emotions, their 'old wives' tales', and the passion of birth-giving. The aim is to transform labour and delivery into efficiently organised medical processes, without the intrusion of those psychosexual elements that threaten the smooth running of the medical system. Admittedly, these psychological elements in childbirth are today briefly acknowledged, but only when expressed in the language of consumerism.

Much of the work of the obstetrician is directed towards the formulation of diagnoses of pathology, provisional or definitive. In practice, many of these diagnoses are incorrect. They are termed 'false positives'. It is often taken for granted that it is better to make a false positive diagnosis – of a possible low-lying placenta, intrauterine growth retardation or cephalo-pelvic disproportion, for example – than to miss a diagnosis that should have been made. This assumption fails to take into the reckoning the harm that false positives can do. They result in anxiety for the woman – and to a lesser extent for all concerned – and lead to unjustified obstetric intervention. The striving to diagnose, often in the face of insufficient evidence, the concern to reveal the pathological, to pinpoint malfunction, is itself a disease.

The outcome of assessing a woman entirely in terms of the projected obstetric performance of her pelvis, of estimating the events of pregnancy and birth exclusively in terms of risk, is that many women come to be labelled 'high–risk'; their pregnancy is treated as abnormal, they feel set apart and often, even in early pregnancy, defective and inadequate, and they lose confidence in their bodies. This may be compounded by iatrogenic intervention which causes further breakdown in the normal physiological process of childbirth.

Illich observes, 'Diagnosis always intensifies stress, defines incapacity, imposes inactivity, and focuses apprehension on nonrecovery, on uncertainty, and on one's dependence on future medical findings, all of which amounts to a loss of autonomy or self-definition.'[20]

The midwife must be able to diagnose deviations from the normal, to intervene, and to refer to the obstetrician when necessary, but her important skills are in maintaining and supporting the normal physiological processes of birth. In the majority of northern industrial countries today these skills are undervalued. This is equally true in all those countries of the developing world where modern obstetrics has been introduced in the form of gleaming modern hospitals in big cities, often hundreds of miles away from the women they are intended to serve. The media extols each new advance in high-tech medicine, each new technological discovery and 'miracle' revelation, and the needs of the vast majority of mothers and babies, who neither require this technology nor benefit from it, are in danger of being forgotten. It is midwives who can redress the balance. When midwives and women having babies unite to speak out with a clear voice it may be possible at last to achieve a new focus on birth as a major life experience rather than a medical crisis.

MIDWIVES SEEKING CHANGE

There is now a strong movement in midwifery which is questioning accepted obstetric procedures and critically examining all different kinds of intervention, including much traditional intervention by midwives. Increasingly midwives are engaged in research and they are in the forefront of change.

It was a midwife who did research on shaving of the perineum and on the use of enemas in labour and discovered that neither practice contributed towards a sterile perineum, that shaving caused abrasions through which infection could enter, that an enema did not speed the progress of labour, and that both routines caused extreme discomfort.[21]

It was a midwife who conducted a randomised control trial of episiotomy in a study that revealed that episiotomy has no advantages over a second-degree laceration, and that there is less perineal trauma when episiotomy is restricted to those cases in which otherwise a tear into the rectum appears inevitable.[22]

Research is one main theme. Another is direct action for better care in childbirth. The consumer movement of the 1970s and 1980s has created a new awareness and an assertiveness in midwives, who are allying themselves with mothers in demanding change. We have discovered that changes in care which run counter to those of the obstetric establishment come about only when women say what they want and say it loud and clear. Midwives and mothers are working together towards a new childbirth which acknowledges that women should be able to make decisions themselves about their bodies.

Birth is an intensely personal experience. Yet it is more than that: the way we give birth is also a political issue. When women are herded into large hospitals like cattle, when their own choices are disregarded, or they do not even realise that there are any choices; when the natural rhythms of birth are ignored, when they lie on delivery tables like fish on a slab about to be filleted, and are subjected to the crude assault of routine episiotomy – our western form of female genital mutilation – *all* women are abused. And when, after birth, their babies are taken away from them to be put in plastic boxes, while their arms are empty, *all* women are degraded.

There is in midwifery today a new raised consciousness

concerning the unique nature of the midwife's task and of birth as a developmental experience. Midwives realise that they are vital mediators in childbirth. They are acknowledging that they need to act as mediators between obstetricians and women. They must cope with the anxiety of the woman in labour about what 'they' are going to do to her, and also with the anxiety of the obstetrician, and resist unnecessary intervention resulting from this. This puts midwives under a great deal of stress, but now that they are talking openly about it, and sharing their experiences, they can begin to work out strategies to deal with these situations.

From an anthropological point of view, midwives have always been mediators between nature and culture. They deal with blood and body fluids, and with the human being at its first raw, elemental moment of existence. They have to be able to understand feelings which are passionate and basic. They are witnesses to the first reaching-out of arms towards the newborn which lies at the root of human love and, because it expresses the bonding of family members, is the essence of social organisation. In childbirth midwives touch the two worlds of the instinctual and the cultural, bringing them into harmony. Such a calling requires not domination and control, but careful observation and sensitive awareness. It needs patience and a willingness to wait for the unfolding of life. It requires skill in helping the labouring woman to have confidence in herself and the power of her uterus.

The new midwifery has a vital part to play in the women's movement and is at the very centre of the great creative upheaval which is taking place as we reclaim our bodies and come to learn about, understand and glory in them. This new midwifery gives vivid expression to the way in which women are discovering strength and sisterhood as we turn to help and support one another during the intense, exhilarating and powerful experience of childbirth.

NOTES

1   The Tao Te Ching. This particular translation is from John Heider, *The Tao of Leadership*, Wildwood House, 1986.

2   Mary Chamberlain, *Old Wives' Tales*, Virago, 1981; Jean Donnison, *Midwives and Medical Men*, Heinemann, 1977.

3   Jean Donnison, 'The development of the occupation of midwife; a comparative view', *Midwifery is a Labour of Love*, Maternal Health Society, 1981, pp. 38–52.

4   Jean Towler and Joan Bramall, *Midwives in History and Society*, Croom Helm, 1986, p. 125.

5   Alice Clark, *Working Life of Women in the Seventeenth Century*, Routledge, 1982, quoted in Margaret Connor Versluysen, 'Old wives' tales? Women healers in English history', in Celia Davies (ed.), *Rewriting Nursing History*, Croom Helm, 1980.

6   Mary Chamberlain, op. cit.

7   R. White, *Social Change and the Development of the Nursing Profession*, Kimpton, 1978.

8   Irvine Loudon, personal communication, and Irvine Loudon, 'Puerperal fever, the strephococcus and the sulphonamides, 1911–1945', *British Medical Journal*, vol. 295, 1987, pp. 485–9.

9   G. Geddes, *Puerperal Septicaemia: Its Causation, Symptoms, Prevention and Treatment*, John Wright, 1912.

10 Elizabeth Davies, *Heart and Hands: A Guide For Midwifery*, John Monroe, 1981.

11 A. Mangay Maglaceas and John Simons, 'The potential of the traditional birth attendant', *WHO Offset Publication*, no. 95, 1986, in *Childbirth Alternatives Quarterly*, vol. 8, no. 3, Spring 1987, p. 12.

12 J. Garcia, S. Garforth and S. Ayers, 'Midwives confined? Labour ward policies and routines', in A. Thomson and S. Robinson (eds), *Research and the Midwife Conference Proceedings*, King's College, London, 1985; 'Royal College of Midwives' Evidence of the Review Body for Nursing Staff, Midwives, Health Visitors and Professions Allied to Medicine for 1987', *Midwives' Chronicle*, vol. 100 (supplement), 1986, pp. 1–39; Editorial, 'Midwives of the future', *Lancet*, vol. 1, 1987, pp. 664–6.

13 Mavis Kirkham, 'A feminist perspective in midwifery', in C. Webb (ed.), *Feminist Practice in Women's Health Care*, John Wiley, 1986.

14 Mavis Kirkham, op. cit., pp. 35–50.

15 Mavis Kirkham, op. cit.

16 Figures for Italy, the Netherlands and Denmark from Statistical Office of European Communities, *Demographic Statistics*; figures for Finland, Sweden and the USA from United Nations, *Demographic Yearbook*.

17 B.M. Morgan, C.J. Bulpitt, P. Clifton and P.J. Lewis, 'The consumer attitude to obstetric care', *British Journal of Obstetrics and Gynaecology*, vol. 90, 1984, pp. 624–8; S. William, M. Hepburn and

C. McIlwaine, 'Consumer view of epidural analgesia', *Midwifery*, vol. 1, 1985, pp. 32–6.

18 Michael Klein, Ivor Lloyd, Christopher Redman, Michael Bull and A.C. Turnbull, 'A comparison of low-risk pregnant women booked for delivery in two systems of care: shared-care (consultant) and integrated general practice unit', Parts I and II, *British Journal of Obstetrics and Gynaecology*, vol. 90, 1983, pp. 118–28.

19 From the testimony of Sally Tom of the American College of Nurse-Midwives in *Nurse Midwifery: Consumers' Freedom of Choice. Hearing Before Subcommittee on Oversight and Investigations of the Committee on Interstate and Foreign Commerce*. House of Representatives, 18 December 1980.

20 Ivan Illich, *Medical Nemesis: The Expropriation of Health*, Pantheon Books, 1976.

21 Mona L. Romney, 'Pre-delivery shaving: an unjustified assault?', *Journal of Obstetrics and Gynaecology*, vol. 1, 1980, pp. 33–5; Mona L. Romney and H. Gordon, 'Is your enema really necessary?', *British Medical Journal*, vol. 282, 1981, pp. 1269–71.

22 Jenny Sleep *et al.*, 'West Berkshire perineal management trial', *British Medical Journal*, vol. 289, 1984, pp. 507–90.

INTRODUCTION

BRITAIN

Since the Second World War midwifery in Britain has been eroded. A study commissioned by the Department of Health and Social Security in 1985 revealed a duplication of resources provided by midwives and general practitioners.[1] Ninety-one per cent of hospital midwives and 66 per cent of community midwives work in antenatal clinics where they cannot use their skills, and instead are employed as receptionists, assistants to the doctor, or chaperones.

Because increasing numbers of women have gone into hospital to give birth community midwives have assisted at fewer deliveries. In 1960 each midwife was responsible for fifty-six deliveries during the year, whereas by 1979 she was responsible for only three.

In hospital high rates of obstetric intervention in normal childbirth, including Caesarean section, are associated with an increase in autocratic decision-making by doctors about care. Midwives are given orders and may only be allowed to make the most trivial decisions. Unit policy, rather than knowledge of the individual woman and clinical skill, determines decision-making. Sixty-five per cent of midwives in teaching hospitals, for example, say that policy regulates when they carry out vaginal examinations. Thus midwives are prevented from developing confidence in making their own decisions about the conduct of labour. Postnatally there is duplication of the work of doctors and midwives, too, and midwives are prevented from making basic decisions about how they look after mothers and babies. More than 80 per cent of midwives reveal that in their hospitals a doctor has to decide whether a mother and baby are fit enough to go home.

In this chapter Caroline Flint, a midwife researcher and activist, explains how this has happened, and makes proposals for urgent change in the way midwives work.

NOTE

1 Sarah Robinson, 'Responsibilities of midwives and medical staff', *Midwives' Chronicle*, March 1985, pp. 64–70.

ON THE BRINK: MIDWIFERY IN BRITAIN

CAROLINE FLINT

In the beginning, there were women and men and babies, and midwives. Midwifery has to be the oldest profession: at the beginning of this century there were three specific professional groups – lawyers, doctors and midwives. The Professions Supplementary to Medicine Act was not passed until 1960. The Nurses Act was passed in 1919, whereas the Midwives Act which laid down regulations for the education and practice of midwifery, and resulted in the Central Midwives Board, was passed in 1902.

Midwifery in Britain is currently in a state of crisis. On the one hand there are women clamouring for a more gentle, normal way of birth, for respect and acknowledgment that it is *their* birth, *their* baby, *their* body and that the experience of that birth will affect them for the rest of their lives. On the other hand there are the obstetricians who in their powerful and self-confident way are saying, 'This is dangerous, we need to control it. This is scientific, we need to be in charge.' The ordinary midwife looks around for allies; she turns to her colleagues but they are silent. When she pleads with them they turn their backs – they feel threatened, oppressed, they are keeping their noses clean, they are keeping quiet. An oppressed group turns in upon itself: 'You should just shut up and get on with your job, after all that's all this is – a job, like anyone else's – and you don't want to lose it.' The midwife knows that this isn't *just a job*. She knows that her actions today and her words tomorrow will affect a woman for ever, will turn a girl into a mother, a lad into a father and two diverse people into someone's parents. She knows that her words and her actions will travel down through time: 'Well, when your

Granny had Alison the midwife said . . .'. The midwife knows that she is involved in one of the most significant events that ever happen to a human being and that somehow *it isn't right* that women are being tricked and deceived, made to do things that aren't right for them, forced to adopt a role which is not appropriate for them.

She turns to senior midwives. They must know, they've been around a long time and must be able to see what is happening to women; they might even have experience of better things, of other ways. But the senior midwives turn away from her, saying, 'Childbirth is dangerous. We need to be in control of it. We need to contain it. We must listen to the obstetricians. They know best.' She realises that these women have been alienated and isolated from their colleagues, and that they are alone in their hierarchical posts. They haven't talked with a woman going through childbirth for a long time, they haven't examined a woman, advised a woman, listened to a woman, or supported a woman going through the throes of labour for many years; they feel out of touch with women, out of touch with other midwives, they have allied themselves with the obstetricians because they are the people they meet most often and they are the people who have most power and influence. These obstetricians are usually male, middle class, beautifully dressed, and often extremely attractive; they smell nice, are carefully manicured, wealthy, powerful, successful and well-spoken. No wonder the (invariably) female senior midwife allies herself with these glorious beings. They are more attractive to her than her own kind.

The midwife turns to the women she cares for. Here at last is someone who feels the same as she does – but her contact with each woman is so short that it is almost impossible to build up a meaningful relationship. She rarely has time to actually talk with a woman; she reels away feeling frustrated and very much alone.[1] Where can the ordinary midwife turn?

The midwife looks around to see how midwives practise and she sees enormous disparity: in some places midwives practise to their full potential, supported by their midwife managers and supervisors of midwives, working as colleagues with their fellow medical professionals; in other places midwives are midwives in name only, and their every action is dictated by the doctors in the form of 'policy'. The midwife's role is to support women through interventions which she may or may not believe are appropriate for this particular woman. The role for which she has been trained and prepared doesn't exist, and to cope with this situation she has two alternatives: to fight and try to achieve change, and then to retire wounded and crushed and leave the profession when she can no longer bear fighting against the odds, or she can accept that she cannot change it, become passive and sublimate her feelings, an efficient operator under the situation as it is, and challenge nothing, 'just do her job'. She then finds it very hard when women challenge what is being done to them because it stirs in her painful memories of how she felt when she first came to this place. Now that she has justified what is happening to herself she finds it just too difficult when someone else challenges it. It is too painful for her to take on the role of being 'with woman'. Instead she turns away from women and becomes 'with doctor', or even 'with policy' because often the doctor who instigated the policy has long gone and there is no rational reason behind it in the light of more up-to-date research.

AN OVERVIEW

Throughout the UK midwives are subjected to petty tyrannies from their superiors. They receive abysmally low salaries. They are subject to the orders of their supervisors, most of whom have never even seen a woman in labour during the past five years, are often woefully out of date with regard to clinical thinking, and frequently confuse their correct role with that of the disciplinarian. Those who see their role as that of supporter, guide and mentor are rare. It has to be said that this behaviour which seems, and is, so destructive is probably only to be expected. A threatened group turns in upon itself. Each midwife is aware that she is the last of her line, because she is so poorly paid; and because she works in an environment in which the shortage of staff frequently verges on the unsafe she is exhausted most of the time, unable to take part in political action to strengthen her profession and too tired to go to meetings or to take on any extra commitment, even though she knows it is important for her profession. Senior midwives bully their subordinates because they are isolated and alienated both from other midwives and from women. They are also involved in an impossible job; they work in a hierarchy which was designed for the army and adapted for nurses, and the thread running through the structure is that the person at the bottom of the pile will obey orders. It is questionable whether this philosophy works for nurses, but it most certainly doesn't work for midwives, who need to be able to be strong and flexible, and to adapt their care to a particular woman, labour, and pregnancy, which is different from any other labour or pregnancy that has ever been. Midwives need to be extraordinarily adaptable; instant obedience really doesn't fit in with these requirements, and when a midwife works in a system geared for this it puts enormous pressure on her.

The senior midwife in the National Health Service is working in an impossible way. Unlike her medical colleagues she has completely left clinical practice. Even the Professor of Obstetrics does the occasional Caesarean section and a regular antenatal clinic; he keeps in physical contact with women going through childbirth, hears what they say, how they feel; he is in touch with his roots, the reason that he is here. She is out of touch with women, except for the letters of complaint or praise that she receives and the occasional chat she has with representatives of the consumer groups. She is also out of touch with clinical practice. Her job is such that she is kept ridiculously busy; often the Director of Midwifery Services will have anything up to fifteen meetings that she has to attend in one week. She is invariably the lone midwife at each meeting, fighting against other vested interests for the midwifery service and for the needs of women. When she has done all that, is it any wonder that she can't bring herself to go to other meetings where she would learn more clinically? Often the days of clinical practice seem to her very distant, and so when she meets a midwife whom she finds difficult to cope with or who is disturbing the peace of her maternity unit, she can often challenge that midwife's clinical practice with the full knowledge that she will be backed up by the Health Authority, who are always loath to challenge any of the managers they have appointed, and by the doctors, who have to work with her for the foreseeable future and don't particularly want midwives practising their skills fully because this challenges their own practice.

Midwives feel oppressed and threatened. They are at the

bottom of the pile as far as status and salary are concerned. Their influence is minimal. There is no one on whom to blame this feeling of discomfort but themselves. Time and time again at Royal College of Midwives' Annual Meetings the delegates say, 'It is our own fault, we are our own worst enemies, it is up to us to stand up and be counted, it is up to each one of us to take our profession forward.' In many ways this is true, but it is understandable that most midwives feel impotent when they try to change and improve maternity care.

The other result of the midwifery profession being oppressed and inward-looking is that women having babies come even lower in the pecking order than midwives, and at a very vulnerable time in their lives can be subjected to petty tyrannies. Problems in the midwifery profession are acted out upon them. Allied to this is the difficulty that the midwife looking after the woman invariably doesn't know that woman and has not been able to build up a relationship with her, because the pattern of maternity care in the United Kingdom ensures that she meets different midwives in the antenatal clinic each time she visits it. The midwives who work in the antenatal clinic and the midwife she may meet at her GP's surgery are different from the midwives who work in the labour ward, so that when she is in labour she is attended by total strangers, and if her labour is of normal length it is likely that she will have two or three staff changes during the time of her labour. Then after she has had her baby she goes to the postnatal ward, where she is tended by yet more midwives, and then home again to the care of several community midwives, most of whom she has never met before.

INDEPENDENT MIDWIFERY

In many parts of the country there are independent midwives – midwives who practise outside the National Health Service, who either advertise or find their clients by word of mouth. These midwives book women for delivery at home. They examine the woman, ascertain her full medical history, and send blood for analysis to private haematology laboratories. They approach the woman's GP but if, as is usual, he is not interested in providing medical cover for a home birth, they inform the local supervisor of midwives. It is then up to her, the Supervisor, to find a GP if she can. Often this is not possible, or the GP is not acceptable to the woman. The independent midwife breathes a sigh of relief, because if an emergency arises she would much prefer either to transfer the woman to hospital, where there are doctors who spend their lives practising obstetrics, or to summon the obstetric 'flying squad' in the knowledge that proficient obstetricians will arrive, rather than to put up with a GP who is in essence another midwife (but usually with less midwifery experience) and who may not be able to offer any constructive help in an emergency. Having said that, there are a few GPs who have kept their skills in home births, who have consistently supported women in their desire to have their babies at home and who provide much support and expertise to both women and midwives.

The independent midwife can care for a woman throughout pregnancy, labour and birth. Her obligations are to notify the local supervisor of midwives of her intention to practise and to refer the woman or her baby to a doctor in the case of any illness or abnormality of the mother, foetus or baby. Her other legal obligation is to notify the local Health Authority of the birth of the baby within thirty-six hours of the child being born. Often the woman only sees a doctor if there is cause for alarm.

The independent midwife truly practises as a midwife. She takes responsibility for all her practice and provides continuity of care for each woman. This means that the mother has the same person (or the same couple if the midwife works with a partner, as many do) throughout her pregnancy, labour and puerperium. The other midwives who practise their art fully are those who work in hospitals where, because of supportive midwifery management, they are able to fulfil their role and where the doctors don't expect to take over or even interrupt the labouring woman unless asked. This happens in few hospitals. It happens more frequently in a two-tier unit, where there are no obstetric registrars and the midwives refer directly to the consultant obstetricians (as suggested in the 'Short' Report of 1980).[2] It also happens in one private maternity hospital where the obstetricians rely greatly on the midwives.

Legally women are able to choose to have a baby at home anywhere in the United Kingdom, and recent evidence has shown that this is a safe option for many women,[3] but in practice in many areas it is virtually impossible for a woman to have a baby at home unless she is extremely articulate and emotionally very strong. Most women at this time feel weak and easily intimidated and often it is quite a battle to secure a home birth. The woman first goes to see her GP, and when she tells her/him that she would like to have her baby at home she is given an emotionally charged lecture along the lines of, 'I wouldn't allow my wife to have a baby at home. You are risking your baby's life. I shall wash my hands of you.' Usually, she is completely taken aback by the doctor's emotional response to the idea of home birth; if her partner or family also discourages her she is likely to take her 'referral letter' to the GP's preferred hospital and try to forget that she had ever entertained the idea of having her baby at home.

However, if she is still determined she may approach a midwife, either someone she meets in the hospital antenatal clinic or a community midwife. The midwife may also interrogate her: 'There are no GPs in this area who will attend home births' (although midwives should know that the attendance of a doctor is unnecessary in a normal labour); 'We don't do many home births – we are out of practice.' If she is lucky she may meet a midwife who greets the suggestion of a home birth with pleasure and encouragement. Here, however, she may well encounter another facet of having a baby at home; she may find that the midwife who takes on a home birth is herself harassed and bullied, often by her superiors, who don't allow her to stay 'on call' for a woman she has got to know during pregnancy.

One experienced midwife was strictly forbidden by her senior midwife from coming into the hospital to deliver when she wasn't on call. The midwife felt too intimidated to disobey; instead, she persuaded many of the women who wanted to be delivered by her in hospital to have their babies at home where she could go to them when they were in labour even if she wasn't officially on call. As she said,

'I can only deliver in hospital when I am on duty, so other midwives deliver my patients, but immediately after the birth they are mine again and I have the three evening visits to do. On the other hand, when I deliver someone else's patient and am up all night, having already worked eleven hours during the day, the senior midwife rings me up at 4 p.m. telling me to do the evening visit because I believe in continuity of care. I could choke her because I feel so tired, but the only answer is to leave if you can't cope.'[4]

The senior midwife is now intimating that the midwife should not be going out to the women she has booked for home delivery because, 'It isn't fair for you to get all the home deliveries. The other midwives should get a chance.' If this were an isolated incidence of bullying on the part of one senior member of our profession towards another it wouldn't be worth mentioning, but from all over the country I hear of midwives not 'being allowed' to go out to women they have booked when they are not officially 'on call'. This is so obviously against the interests of the women that one wonders whose interests it actually serves. It certainly isn't in the interest of the midwife who is eager and willing to go out to women she has booked because she cares about continuity of care. It obviously isn't in the interest of those midwives who never book anyone for delivery because they have lost confidence in their delivery skills and find it too threatening to be with a woman during labour, to be called to someone they don't know and don't want to deliver. It appears to be petty and spiteful behaviour, often directed against the midwife who still has enthusiasm and love for her profession.

An interesting phenomenon seems to be developing within the midwifery profession in the United Kingdom. The midwifery profession throughout the world is under threat; it is usually threatened by the medical profession and, if not overtly by them, by the 'public prosecutor', but the UK seems to be the only country where midwives are at threat from members of their own profession, the only country where midwives use as a primary recourse the disciplinary system when trying to deal with practitioners who are strong, enthusiastic and outspoken. Midwives are intimidated by use of 'investigation' or 'super-vision' when there is disagreement in ideas about clinical practice or when a midwife is showing signs of being a 'practitioner in her own right'. Although lip service is paid to this concept, when 'practitioners in their own right' actually practise they are soon shot down, as instanced by the period in the early part of 1988 when 30 per cent of the independent midwives in the UK were either being 'investigated', appearing before the Professional Conduct Committee, being 'supervised' closely or being asked to write statements on their practice. All these apparently unrelated events show a punitive trend towards a group of midwives whose intelligence, excellence in standards of practice, and commitment both to their profession and to mothers is renowned.

Women write to say that they have booked for a home delivery because they so much want to have someone with them during labour that they know, only to be told that they will have any one of fourteen midwives who might be there when they deliver. When they complain about the lack of continuity of care they are told, 'Never mind, you'll have a chance to meet them over a cup of tea on the first Wednesday of the month.' The woman goes along to this 'tea party' only to find that it has been cancelled because of pressure of work, or to meet ten of the midwives because the other four have days off or holidays, and when she goes into labour one of those who was on holiday is the midwife who arrives at her door. Even if it is a midwife she has met over a cup of tea, how can anyone make a meaningful relationship with the one who is going to be with them during the most intimate experience a human being goes through, when they are meeting such a large number of midwives?

HOW WE GOT HERE

There has been a tussle between midwives and obstetricians since they first came into existence. The medical establishment was so worried about the midwifery profession that the 1902 Midwives Act was only passed because the Central Midwives Board was to consist of a majority of doctors, and it wasn't until 1973 – seventy-one years after the Act was passed – that a midwife instead of a doctor was made Chairwoman of the Central Midwives Board. Now the Midwifery Committee of the English National Board has one obstetrician in its ranks and the Midwifery Committee of the United Kingdom Central Council has no obstetrician: it is encouraging that midwives are finally ruling themselves. However, it seems sad that mothers are not represented on either of the Midwifery Committees or on the Central Midwives Board.

THE MIDWIFE'S DILEMMA

The midwife is aware of her powerlessness in a hierarchical system but she is also aware of her power: her power over women who are in an extremely vulnerable position and her power over doctors, if she ever uses it. Interestingly, if a midwife actually confronts a doctor, if she shares her knowledge with a doctor or if she takes a doctor under her wing and guides him/her, often she can have a huge influence on his/her future practice. But the most basic power that the midwife has is that she is the person who does the work. Midwives often say, 'The doctor said I must rupture her membranes when she got to four centimetres,' or, 'The policy says that we must rupture the membranes at four centimetres,', but the person who actually ruptures them is the midwife. She is also the person who gives the enema, shaves the pubic hair or performs the vaginal examination every two hours when she doesn't consider that this is either necessary or good practice. The midwife doesn't have to go on strike in order to avoid doing those acts that she finds are contrary to her professional opinion. She just has to say that she considers that this is not a justifiable action, that it is not an ethical action or that, in her professional opinion, it is not a correct action and that she is not doing it. If the consultant wants all 'his' women shaved she will ring him every time one of 'his' women is admitted in order for him to perform the shave.

This is easy to suggest and is obviously more difficult to do. It is even more difficult to do without the support of senior midwives or without the support of colleagues, but it must be said that some midwives are going to have to be brave enough to stand up in this way. They may well be hounded out of their profession, but their sacrifice will be noticed and publicised and will lay the foundations for similar actions which will have the effect of empowering our profession.

When one considers the numbers of midwives who are already leaving the profession (80 per cent do not go on to practise their skills) because of disagreements with their supervisor or their dilemmas over 'policies', it seems very wasteful and destructive. There is an enormous amount of pain involved in these actions. It seems that a more *kamikaze* type of action might well be more productive. If someone within a group which feels as threatened as the midwifery profession wants to initiate changes they have to take on board that they will be hated and hounded, that they will be threatening to other midwives (even, sadly, those from whom they would expect to receive support, who appear to have the same objectives as themselves) and that they need to set up for themselves a support group outside the profession – mothers they have delivered, those they have looked after during pregnancy and postpartum, partners who are as interested in childbirth as themselves. It is not useful for midwives who are being hounded to retire wounded and stay quiet; it is essential that every instance of harassment of midwives is highlighted and publicised.

A perfect example of the power of the media is the case of Wendy Savage, the consultant obstetrician who was suspended for negligence on 24 April 1985 and later exonerated when the whole process used against her was challenged as being irregular.[5] If Wendy had remained quiet she would have been unjustly hounded out of her job, instead of which she has become representative of someone who cares for women and the way they have babies. It has not helped her much: she is aware that she will never again be in a comfortable and cosy position as an obstetrician, and that everything that happens to any of the women she cares for will be questioned, pored over, dissected and discussed; but if she had just shrunk away (which is the normal human reaction to this type of threat) nothing would have changed for women and nothing would have been highlighted. From the media coverage of her case several aspects of childbirth have been brought out into the open.

- The control of childbirth has very little to do with women and either their needs or wants, and often they are like pawns in a power game.
- The medical profession is extremely cruel to its own who dare to step out of line (for 'medical' also read 'midwifery').
- There is no consensus on the way women whose babies present by the breech should be cared for. (There is huge dissension over whether the women concerned should have Caesarean sections or be allowed to deliver vaginally.)
- And, equally, there is no consensus on how *any* woman expecting a baby should be cared for.

- Women care deeply about the way they give birth and about those who champion and acknowledge that desire. (Thousands of people marched in support of Wendy on two occasions during her ordeals.)
- The use of disciplinary hearings solves almost nothing, but simply causes great pain to both the discipliner and the disciplined. The state of the Obstetrics Department at the London and Mile End Hospitals since the hearing and Wendy Savage's reinstatement is certainly no better, and probably even worse, than it was before her suspension. All those midwives who have been subjected to disciplinary hearings will know that afterwards, even if they win their case, the atmosphere is so strained and they are treated so much as lepers, that nothing is or can ever be the same again. Comfort and innocence have gone, only pain remains, to become a dull ache and, finally, a sad memory, bringing a deeper compassion for others in the same predicament and an ability to see more widely than before.

THE MAJOR INFLUENCES

In 1975 a programme in the *Horizon* series on television highlighted the state of childbirth in the United Kingdom.[6] It showed that a large number of women's labours were being induced and accelerated. Shortly afterwards an article in the *Sunday Times* by Louise and Oliver Gillie picked up the same theme and the nation was alerted to what was happening to women.[7] A survey of 2,000 women by Sheila Kitzinger, for the National Childbirth Trust,[8] showed that women who had their labours induced frequently needed more analgesia during the labour, were more likely to have an instrumental delivery, and their babies were more likely to need extra resuscitation and to go to the Special Care Baby Unit than their counterparts whose labours were not induced. Then in 1979 Sheila Kitzinger published *The Good Birth Guide*.[9] This caused uproar within the maternity services: who did she think she was? She, who wasn't even a midwife, what trouble was she causing? What desires was she stirring up in women coming to St Freda's only to discover that she had given St Freda's very low ratings and that St Megan's down the road had a flexible policy on the positions women could take up during labour, that their induction rate was very low and that the midwives were very kind and listened to what women were saying to them? For the first time, hospitals were brought face to face with the fact that they were providing a service, that those who were receiving that service were not always impressed with it, and that the recipients of the service actually wanted something different from what the service providers had been trying to provide. The revolution had begun.

In February 1982, in response to an instruction from a London hospital obstetrician that women in his unit were not to deliver in alternative positions until it had been proved safer than the 'conventional' position, 5,000 women and their partners demonstrated outside the hospital and then went on to hold a celebration of childbirth on Parliament Hill Fields. Following on from that, two 'Active Birth Conferences' were held in Wembley Conference Centre, the first in October 1982 and then, because it was so overbooked, another in March 1983. The National Childbirth Trust, a consumer group dedicated to 'education for parenthood' which had been founded in 1956, was the 'mother' of many of the events that happened at this time, although it had adopted a policy of a softly softly approach, designed not to antagonise but to change and improve through cooperation with senior midwives and obstetricians. Its influence was obvious: Sheila Kitzinger was and is an NCT teacher and tutor; Janet Balaskas was an NCT teacher before founding the Active Birth Movement; many of the parents who demonstrated outside the Royal Free Hospital had come with other members of their local NCT branches.

In 1976 a group of student midwives met and aired their frustrations at the level of midwifery training they were receiving and at what was happening to women, who were generally being treated as 'patients' with a pathological condition, and who received medical care which was geared to a labour that 'could only be considered normal in retrospect'. The Central Midwives Board had also expressed concern at this in their booklet entitled *The Role of the Midwife*.[10] It appears to be readily acknowledged that the midwife is responsible for the care of normal childbirth, but perhaps one of the main threats to the execution of that role is the practical application of the philosophy that childbirth is only normal in retrospect. When this philosophy is adopted by those caring for a woman in a delicately balanced state and who is experiencing pain, it has a profound effect on the outcome of labour. If the midwife who is with the woman at this vulnerable time believes that she is capable of coping with her labour and that her body is designed to work well in labour and produce a live, healthy baby, that the uterus will contract efficiently, that the cervix will open (because that is what it was designed to do, wasn't it?), that the baby will be fine, that what is happening is normal and good and is experienced by women all over the world, she is obviously alert to any deviations from the norm. She doesn't expect them to happen, and they usually don't. On the other hand, if labour is looked upon as a dangerous and potentially lethal condition, the uterus seen as inefficient, the mother's body as menacing to the baby, the whole process becomes potentially abnormal, and fear is generated – fear amongst the doctors, fear amongst the midwives, fear within the mother and father. Fear affects labour; mammals who are afraid cannot labour smoothly. Fear inhibits the physiological process of labour; it increases perception of pain so that the woman needs more analgesia, more 'help' to accelerate the labour and the baby becomes distressed. Electronic foetal monitoring is all part of the same fearful philosophy that the mother's body could have the effect of abruptly terminating the baby's life.

The student midwives who met in 1976 formed the Association of Radical Midwives.[11] Its aims are:

1   To re-establish the confidence of the midwife in her own skills.
2   To share ideas, skills and information.
3   To encourage midwives in their support of a woman's active participation in childbirth.
4   To reaffirm the need for midwives to provide continuity of care.
5   To explore alternative patterns of care.
6   To encourage evaluation of development in our field.

The Association of Radical Midwives is committed to the origins of the name 'midwife', the Old English meaning of which is 'with woman'. The Association seeks to ally itself with women, seeing the midwife and the childbearing woman as intertwined with each other, needing each other and needing each other's support.

The Midwives Information and Resource Service (MIDIRS)[12] was established in 1985, an organisation committed to meeting the midwives' need for information on both clinical research and the political influences important to their profession. The emergence of MIDIRS has increased the midwives' awareness of their role and of their own needs as well as those of the childbearing women. Knowledge makes midwives stronger and more assertive.

The Royal College of Midwives,[13] which has been in existence for much longer than the other organisations and is bigger and more widely consulted, celebrated its centenary in 1981. It is the professional body for midwives and its trades union has concentrated on midwives, their status and professional role: it has defended midwives in trouble both with their employer and professional bodies; it has negotiated for higher salaries for midwives and it has tried to represent the midwife and her point of view. This emphasis on the midwife sometimes appears to leave out mothers, the women who are at the very root of all the discussions, plans, schemes and ideas for the future and about the role of the midwife. This may be because the greater part of the Council of the Royal College of Midwives has been made up of midwifery managers whose only experience of management is within the Health Service. Equally, many of the posts within the College itself are reserved for those 'experienced in management'. The experience of 'management' is valuable and often necessary but, because it is all from one mould, it restricts the variety of approach and the width of vision. Also, it often restricts the personnel to those who have not been through the experience of childbirth. This does not necessarily matter – many of the most sympathetic and sensitive midwives have not experienced childbirth – but it does mean that a huge and life-changing experience which affects all the women with whom midwives come into contact is not represented by those who are deciding policy and future planning for the midwifery profession, so that policies can appear to be divorced from the needs of those they are designed to serve.

The Royal College of Midwives, as is the case with many

professional organisations, has also been slow to catch up on the importance of the media, to realise that the General Secretary of the Royal College of Midwives should be a household name for women everywhere, for she has far more importance in their lives than the General Secretary of the National Union of Mineworkers or the General Secretary of the printers union, whose names they usually know already because of their high media profile.

The other encouraging development from the English National Board for Nursing, Midwifery and Health Visiting, the Association of Radical Midwives and the Royal College of Midwives is the push towards the opening up of more 'direct entry' training schools where women who have not had nursing training can train to be midwives. (It is a longer training than that of State Registered Nurses.) This facet of midwifery training is not new in the United Kingdom and is common in Europe, but in the UK it had died out as the training had lengthened, until only one school remained, in Derby. The advantage of direct-entry training for midwifery is that women are not perceived to be ill when they have a baby. They are seen as going through a normal body state and, therefore, the skills of the nurse in nursing the sick and caring for the helpless are inappropriate. Likewise, the nurse's obedience in the face of directives from the doctor may be unsuitable, for the childbearing woman needs her midwife to be strong and 'with' her – on her side, her advocate and supporter. The other perceived advantage of direct entry midwifery is that many women are inspired by their own childbirth experience and want to help other women to experience a magical time when their baby is born. These women will be more mature, stronger and more articulate, and should exert a very strengthening influence on our profession.

The future lies in an alliance between mothers and midwives. For a long time mothers have been saying that they want (and need) to get to know the midwife or midwives who will be with them throughout their pregnancy, labour and puerperium.[14] To have strangers involved at a time of such intimacy is anathema. Midwives have been saying for years that they want to practise their role fully, that they want to take responsibility for the care of women going through a normal physiological phenomenon. The report published by the National Perinatal Epidemiology

Unit on home birth and its safety echoes an increasing commitment to home birth even from such organisations as the Royal College of Midwives, which in the past has reflected the view of the 760 obstetricians in this country who have deflected women from having their babies at home. When women have their babies at home the woman is in charge. It is her home, she is the hostess and the relationship between the mother and midwife is an equal one; the midwife is truly 'with woman' in her own habitat. The Association of Radical Midwives has published a future plan for maternity care called *The Vision*[15] which describes midwives working in small teams, responsible for a specific number of pregnant women, able to get to know each woman in a meaningful way. Similar aims are reflected in the Royal College of Midwives document *The Role and Education of the Future Midwife in the United Kingdom*.[16] The idea has come of age: the midwife and the woman are both feeling the same, and increasingly each is hearing what the other is saying. Soon their alliance will become strong and by sheer numerical force alone (32,000 practising midwives and 650,000 women having babies every year in England and Wales), they will reclaim birth and their bodies for themselves.

NOTES

1 Menzies, Isabel E.P., 'The functioning of social systems as a defence against anxiety', Tavistock Institute of Human Relations (Belsize Lane, London NW3 5BA), 1970.

2 Green, Josephine, Kitzinger, Jenny and Coupland, Vanessa, 'The division of labour', Childcare and Development Group, University of Cambridge, 1986; 'Second Report from the Social Services Committee. Session (1979–80), Perinatal and Neonatal Mortality', HMSO, 19 June 1980 (the Short Report).

3 Campbell, Rona and MacFarlane, Alison, 'Where to be born – the debate and the evidence', National Perinatal Epidemiology Unit, Oxford, 1987.

4 Personal communication.

5 Savage, Wendy, *A Savage Enquiry: Who Controls Childbirth?* Virago, 1986.

6 'A time to be born', *Horizon*, BBC TV, January 1975.

7 Gillie, Louise and Oliver, 'The childbirth revolution', 13 October 1974, 'The vital first hours', 20 October 1974, *Sunday Times Weekly Review*.

8 Kitzinger, Sheila, 'Some mothers' experiences of induced labour. Submission to the Department of Health and Social Security', National Childbirth Trust, 1975 and 1978.

9 Kitzinger, Sheila, *The Good Birth Guide*, Penguin, 1979.

10 Central Midwives Board, Central Midwives Board for Scotland, Northern Ireland Council for Nurses and Midwives and An Bord Altranais, *The Role of the Midwife*, 1983.

11 Association of Radical Midwives, 62 Greetby Hill, Ormskirk, Lancs, L39 2DT.

12 Midwives' Information and Resource Service, Westminster Hospital, Dean Ryle Street, London SW1 2AP.

13 The Royal College of Midwives, 15 Mansfield Street, London W1M 0BE.

14 Micklethwait, P., Beard, R. and Shaw, Kathleen, 'Expectations of a pregnant woman in relation to her treatment', *British Medical Journal*, vol. 2, 1978, pp. 188–91.

15 Association of Radical Midwives, *The Vision: Proposals for the Future of the Maternity Services*, ARM, 1986.

16 Royal College of Midwives, *Report of the Royal College of Midwives on the Role and Education of the Future Midwife in the United Kingdom*, RCM, 1987.

INTRODUCTION

USA

In the USA less than 5 per cent of births are midwife-attended. This figure is artificially low because in some states where midwifery is illegal the father must sign the birth certificate. Yet even bearing this in mind, it is clear that only a tiny minority of American women are cared for by midwives.

Basically three kinds of midwives exist. There is the certified nurse-midwife (CNM) who is a nurse with subsequent training in midwifery. She works in collaboration with obstetricians and usually practises in a hospital or birth centre. Only 4 per cent of nurse-midwife births take place at home. When a woman is cared for by a CNM she can get Medicaid insurance re-imbursement. Then there is the midwife who has not come into midwifery from a background of nursing but has learned midwifery by apprenticeship to an experienced midwife. She is often described as a 'lay', 'empirical' or 'independent' midwife. The third kind is the 'direct-entry' midwife. She is not a nurse either but has received professional training, including theory and practical experience, and has had to pass a qualifying examination. All these non-nurse midwives care for mothers mainly in the women's own homes with obstetric back-up agreed with one or more physicians so that they can get hospital admission if necessary. They do not usually practise in hospital, though they may work in a birth centre.

In the 1970s it was largely people who chose alternative lifestyles who sought midwife-attended births. In the 1980s a cross-section of the propulation seek midwife care, many of them college-educated with professional careers.

American midwives have two organisations: The American College of Nurse-Midwives and the Midwives' Alliance of North America. The latter includes certified nurse-midwives, empirical midwives and direct-entry midwives who have, like their counterparts in Europe, pursued a course in midwifery at a recognised institution.

Midwifery projects initiated in the 1970s and 1980s have produced overwhelming evidence of the advantages of midwife care for both babies and mothers. When the University of Mississippi Medical Center began a nurse-midwifery service the infant mortality rate was reduced from 39 per 1,000 to 21 per 1,000 within three years. At Stanford University Medical School midwife care resulted in a drop in the episiotomy rate from 73 per cent to 7 per cent. In 287 home births attended by empirical midwives in the Santa Cruz area infant mortality was 3 per 1,000, compared with 15 per 1,000 for the general population in that part of California. In a rural hospital in California the rate was reduced from 24 per 1,000 to 10 per 1,000 with nurse-midwife care. When the programme was ended, it went back to 24 per 1,000. In Texas, at a free-standing birth centre in Raymondville, twenty-five miles from the nearest hospital, where the Family Clinic provides midwife care, the rates of pre-term and low birth weight babies are less than half of those of Texas and of the USA as a whole.

It is with this kind of research in mind that the authors of the next two chapters write about the development of empirical midwifery and direct-entry midwifery in the USA.

Ina May Gaskin has pioneered midwifery at the Farm in Tennessee, where the Home Birth Delivery Service has achieved an infant mortality rate as low as 8.6 per 1,000 compared with 26 per 1,000 for the state of Tennessee. Jo Anne Myers-Ciecko is Academic Director of the Seattle Midwifery School, which offers a three-year direct-entry training programme and continuing education programmes for practising midwives.

MIDWIFERY RE-INVENTED

INA MAY GASKIN

When Alexis de Tocqueville visited the United States in 1831, he commented, 'it [the general equality of condition] creates opinions, gives birth to new sentiments, founds novel customs, and modifies whatever it does not produce.'[1] Although de Tocqueville's observation did not apply to midwifery in the United States in the early nineteenth century, one hundred years later, it fitted perfectly. By 1930, the United States had taken the unique and drastic step of virtually obliterating the profession of midwifery. Except in those isolated and rural areas where traditional midwives and family doctors still cooperated, women no longer had the power to make significant decisions about childbirth. Men, usually doctors, wrote the books and the magazine articles that told women how to think about childbirth: what was safe and what was not. Birth took place in hospitals, planned and administered by men. Doctors delivered babies, and only men, with a very few exceptions, were doctors. Nurses were women, and spent time with laboring mothers, but they did not lay hands on the baby at the most critical moment of the process, the actual birth, nor did they provide the knowledge which underlay the procedures and policies that were carried out in delivery rooms.

By the 1920s, the United States had founded a truly novel custom: that of sanctioning men to make the rules and supply the knowledge for an intimately physical process that they never experienced. Lost totally to the general public was the idea that a woman could be trained to safely attend another woman in labor. With no group of women equal in power to the doctors and thus able to exert a mitigating influence on male-designed policies, childbirth became mechanized, systematized, and regulated. Looking back from the perspective of the 1980s, we see that American women have been subjected, *en masse*, to a variety of extreme, often dangerous procedures in the years since the 1930s, including the use of scopalomine during labor, the prescription of diuretics during pregnancy to control weight, the prescription of cancer-causing DES to mothers during pregnancy, the routine use of forceps for first-time mothers, and now, in the 1980s, a national caesarean section rate at a scandalously high 25 per cent. All during the twentieth century, infant mortality rates in the United States have remained higher than those of the other countries of the industrialized world.

Almost certainly in response to the extremity of this situation, a unique kind of midwifery has appeared in the United States, one that runs in two basic streams and has little direct connection with the midwifery it replaced. Because so complete a break in the tradition of midwifery took place in the United States, American women have had to reinvent a profession that many women have decided is essential. The two streams of midwifery (hospital-based nurse-midwifery, and empirical or direct-entry midwifery) developed independently of each other.

Traditional American midwifery was a casualty of a combination of forces peculiar to the colonial history of the United States. Midwives attended all births during the early colonial period. Europeans, as well as the indigenous people of America, kept to the idea that the decision-making power surrounding normal childbirth belonged with women. Birth was seen as a normal, biological process, not as a medical event. While a male physician might be called in the event of an emergency, ordinarily men, whether as husbands or as physicians, did not attend births. Records show that at least one man was prosecuted in the seventeenth century for attending a childbirth.

FROM SOCIAL CHILDBIRTH TO MEDICALIZED CHILDBIRTH

Historians have called the period from the early seventeenth century until the middle of the eighteenth century the period of 'social childbirth'. While birth was regarded as a normal function, it was also recognized that birth could be dangerous and unpredictable. Women gained comfort from one another and took pains to gather together female friends and relatives at the time of birth. Although most midwives of the time had no formal training there were texts of midwifery available in English. Most women knew a lot about childbirth because of the constant network of social exchange surrounding the event. Transmission of knowledge was largely carried out orally and through the apprentice system. We know from diaries and journals of mid-wives of the time that many midwives gathered medicinal plants, applied poultices, prescribed salves, syrups and elixirs, and treated injuries and disease. Midwives also washed and laid out the dead.[2]

The second period of the history of childbirth in America lasted from about 1760 on through the nineteenth century. This period marked the transition between the era of social childbirth and the period of medicalized childbirth, laying the groundwork for the rise of modern obstetrics. It was at the beginning of this second period that male physicians in America began to get involved in childbirth. Many affluent families began to send their sons to European medical schools. One of these young men, William Shippen, Jr, studied the anatomy and physiology of pregnancy in London under William Hunter and sat in on the lectures of William Smellie, the controversial 'man-midwife' who gave instruction in practical midwifery and in the use of obstetrical forceps. Shippen returned to America with the idea that midwifery was a branch of medical science, and he began offering instruction to physicians and midwives.

There began to be an American literature of childbirth written exclusively by male physicians. These texts tended to standardize both practice and attitudes. Later texts usually portrayed mid-wives as incompetent practitioners or ignored them.

The new knowledge of the anatomy and physiology of ges-tation was as revolutionary as were the astronomical investi-gations of the fifteenth century. Once the mysteries of the insides of women began to be revealed, it became much more possible to think of upsetting old values. The use of instruments by male physicians caused a widespread change in attitudes regarding male attendance at birth. Midwives usually did not use forceps, so were at a disadvantage once there began to be competition for who would attend births. Concerns for feelings of mothers were swept aside by the interest in the new technology, which was effective (in the right hands) in helping some labors in which the mother was exhausted while pushing, a problem that formerly was resolved by caesarean section or destruction of the baby in order to save the mother.

Medical schools were on the rise during the nineteenth century, rapidly increasing the supply of male physicians who thought of midwifery as a branch of medicine. With no schools of midwifery, midwives were again at a disadvantage. They had no organizations or network of communications among them, so when physicians began to mount an attack on midwives, they had no effective way to reply, or even to know that they were being systematically attacked. It is significant that there were no midwives who published any objections to their profession being eroded by the medical profession during the years of virulent anti-midwife propaganda. Even before American women began giving birth in hospitals, a large percentage began to choose physicians to attend their births. Choosing a doctor, rather than a midwife, was a way of announcing to the world that you were modern and moving up the social scale. My mother-in-law and her brothers and sisters, born at home in Texas during the early part of this century, all carry as middle names the surname of the doctor who attended their births.

Following the pattern learned from their European counterparts, American physicians began to develop ways to teach obstetrics to medical students by using poor women as teaching material. New surgical techniques and anesthesias were exciting technologies that attracted physicians to work in hospitals. One doctor, Irving Potter of Buffalo, New York, became famous in the 1920s for advocating that the great majority of births be accomplished by the physician reaching into the uterus, turning the baby into a feet-first position, grabbing the feet and pulling the baby out. Many physicians opposed this radical bypass of the natural birth process, probably because so few of them were able to perform the technique and still have a live, uninjured baby.

Joseph DeLee, another famous obstetrician-author of the early half of the century, was so successful in promoting his equally radical ideas that some American women still give birth by the methods he advocated. He argued that the problem with the obstetrics of his time was that too many physicians believed that childbirth was a simple physiologic process.

'Labor has been called, and still is believed by many to be, a normal function,' he stated in 1920. 'Everything, of course, depends on what we define as normal. If a woman falls on a pitchfork and drives the handle through her perineum, we call that pathologic – abnormal, but if a large baby is driven through the pelvic floor, we say that is natural, and therefore normal. If a baby were to have his head caught in a door very lightly, but enough to cause a cerebral hemorrhage, we would say that is decidedly pathogenic, but were a baby's head crushed against a tight pelvic floor, and a hemorrhage in the brain kills it, we call this normal, at least we say that the function is natural, not pathogenic . . . . In fact only a small minority of women escape damage during labor, while 4 per cent of the babies are killed and a large indeterminable number are more or less injured by the direct action of the natural process itself. So frequent are these bad effects that I have often wondered whether Nature did not deliberately intend women should be used up in the process of reproduction, in a manner analogous to that of the salmon, which dies after spawning?'[3]

It may seem incredible that such statements could have been accepted as scientifically valid by the medical community, but apparently they were. DeLee's formula for saving women from Nature was the routine delivery of every baby by forceps. He routinely used narcotics and scopalomine during the first stage of labor, then eliminated the second stage of labor by pulling the baby out with forceps. Placentas were manually extracted, according to DeLee's belief that he was preventing hemorrhage and infection.

The power that a single, incompetent, but charismatic obstetrician could wield was brought home to me when I realized, some fifteen years after the birth of my first child in 1966, that this birth had been choreographed by Joseph DeLee, even though he had long been in his grave. I had done my best to have a birth without anesthesia and forceps, but DeLee, dead, was more powerful than my husband and I were alive. Now, in the 1980s, American women in many areas of the country where there is only one hospital with a maternity ward have even less choice than I had in 1966. In some places like this, the caesarean rate may be over 50 per cent for all birthing women.

It is important to recognize that the American system of maternity care did not take the shape it did because of a male conspiracy of bad men. In my opinion, American obstetrics gradually but relentlessly moved in the direction it did simply because women, as an informed group, had no way to comment on the new technologies and techniques that were being designed for them, their daughters and granddaughters. Had women been involved in this decision-making process, it is likely that the American system would have more closely resembled those of the other industrialized countries, where midwives did have some continuing presence, respect and influence through the early part of the twentieth century. Americans quite early became accustomed to thinking of doctors as gods, of pregnancy as illness, and of laboring women as patients.

One notable example of a physician who achieved god status as early as the nineteenth century was J. Marion Sims. Generally credited with being the world's first gynecological surgeon, he profited by the system of slavery in his surgical experiments in vaginal repair surgery. This man, unlike any of his European counterparts, was able legally to take possession of black women's bodies and to perform surgery on them at his will. He actually bought some of the subjects of his experiments. One woman named Anarcha, who had suffered a vaginal wall injury at childbirth, endured thirty sessions of surgery without anesthesia before Sims was satisfied with the job he had done. Sims became a hero for generations of obstetrician-gynecologists who followed him, many of whom also dreamed of achieving worldwide fame.[4]

In no other country during the early part of the twentieth century did medical men have the unchecked power that American physicians enjoyed. This is not to say that all physicians were power-hungry at that time. The trouble was that the men who most aggressively promoted themselves, in particular the men who wrote for publication in the medical journals, too often turned out to be the ones whose interventive methods became the basis for widespread practice.

At the same time, the rash of anti-midwife propaganda published in the medical journals during the early part of the twentieth century was very effective in persuading physicians all over the country of the necessity of proselytizing against midwifery. Women's magazines of the time promoted the doctors' message, advising pregnant women to go to their doctors with questions about pregnancy, birth and childrearing, never to their female relatives (for fear of being exposed to 'old wives' tales'). So effectively was the women's network of knowledge dismantled that millions of people my age grew up unaware that their own parents had been born at home. Within my own family, it was only when I became a midwife myself that I was able to learn that my great-grandmother had been a midwife, very much respected in her community. She had become an unmentionable person during the years when there was an absolute ban on a positive image of midwives.

Most of the southeastern and southwestern states, because of their rural character and, sometimes, because of the sparseness of their populations, did continue to recognize midwives in a grudging but practical way. Most of these midwives served black or Hispanic women in rural areas, people who did not have much money to spend on maternity or health care. Physicians in such locales would work with the midwives, accepting their emergency cases, happy not to have to cover the routine childbirths for the populations served by the midwives.

THE RISE OF NURSE-MIDWIFERY

Nurse-midwifery had its beginnings in 1918, with the foundation of the Maternity Center Association (MCA) in New York, opened to provide prenatal care in poor neighborhoods and education for mothers. In the early 1930s, the MCA went on to train public health nurses in midwifery, to supervise the remaining immigrant midwives and to attend births among the urban poor and the rural poor in a rural project.[5]

The next organization to foster nurse-midwifery was Mary Breckinridge's Frontier Nursing Service of Kentucky, in 1925. Mary Breckinridge cared for children in devastated postwar France, and while there, admired the French midwives and appreciated the role they played in public health. Once her work in France was over, she decided to seek midwifery training in England and Scotland so she could go back to America and establish a system of midwifery care for poor women in the remote Appalachian region of eastern Kentucky. The area was rugged, accessible only by horse and muleback, and the people lived with no electricity, little transportation, no medical services, and no running water.[6]

Between 1925 and 1941, Breckinridge brought British-trained midwives to work with her or sent Americans to England for training. After the war began, the Frontier Nursing Service, which would more accurately have been named the Frontier Midwifery Service, began training its own nurse-midwives. (One of these midwives was my mother's cousin, a fact I was unaware of until after I became a midwife.) A Metropolitan Life Study of the FNS Midwifery Service of the first 10,000 deliveries between 1925 and 1954 reported that 60 per cent of the births had taken place in the home. Between 1952 and 1954, the FNS rate of premature births was only 37.6 per 1,000 live births, compared with the national average of 76.0 per 1,000 live births. This statistic gives some idea of how a system of individualized midwifery care can reduce the prematurity rate, even in a population that is rightly considered high-risk.

Mary Breckinridge dreamed that other centers like the FNS would spring up to serve rural populations in the United States. It would have been good for the people if this had happened, but midwifery had been too discredited and forgotten to make such a development possible. Besides, not many Americans were aware of the FNS, partly because Mary Breckinridge concentrated on publicizing the service to uppercrust northeastern people who donated funds to the project. The Vanderbilts, Rockefellers and others gave money, but they saw the FNS more as a charity project than as a model of how millions of American women could give birth more safely than they could with the hospital services currently available. After Mary Breckinridge's death, the FNS switched from providing midwifery services for home births to serving as staff for a purely in-hospital midwifery service and educational program.

In 1931, the Lobenstine Midwifery Center, in affiliation with the Maternity Center School of Nurse-Midwifery, began a home delivery service for mothers in New York City, again producing statistics which should have been noticed nationwide.

Twelve years later, the Catholic Maternity Institute was founded in the region of Santa Fe, New Mexico. Their statistics, as well as those of Su Clinica Familiar, a migrant family health clinic estabished in 1972 in the southern tip of Texas, were outstanding.

It was not until 1953 that an American nurse-midwife was officially permitted to attend a birth in a hospital. Two prominent New York obstetricians (Dr Nicholas Eastman and Dr Howard Taylor) arranged for this grand experiment, aware that there were not enough physicians to meet even the minimum demands. The birth rate was high (this was the era before oral contraceptives were introduced), prenatal clinics were swamped, and many mothers gave birth on stretchers in the hallways.

The breakthrough for nurse-midwives came in 1958, when the first school of nurse-midwifery was invited to transfer into a hospital medical center. A tiny group of instructors and students provided care for hundreds of mothers. A couple of other midwifery education programs began in the 1960s, but few people in the United States had any notion of what a nurse-midwife might be. The early graduates of nurse-midwifery schools could not find jobs as midwives because there were none. A study in 1963 showed that of the 535 nurse-midwives in the United States qualified to offer full maternity care, only thirty were actually doing what they had been trained to do. What some of these women did do was to open doors for the midwives who would come later. They attended conferences on childbirth, passed out flyers containing information about midwives, befriended doctors whose minds were not closed, and promoted midwifery whenever and wherever they could. Some of them managed to convince obstetricians to try out working with midwives.

The American College of Nurse-Midwives (ACNM) was formed in 1955, out of nurse-midwives' desire to have their own professional organization. Previous to that time, the only way for nurse-midwives to meet together was at the conventions of the two national nursing organizations, neither of which had developed special sections for nurse-midwives. The ACNM did emphasize, as did the American Nurses Association in 1968, that the nurse-midwife was, first of all, a professional nurse. Nurse-midwifery was defined as 'a clinical specialty in nursing.'

One of the first objectives of the ACNM was to achieve legalization for the nurse-midwife. As of 1969, only two of the fifty states recognized nurse-midwives. ACNM lobbying efforts led to all the other states removing or amending laws which clearly prohibited nurse-midwifery by 1975.

Despite legalization and a policy statement adopted by the American College of Obstetricians and Gynecologists, there was a general reluctance of the medical profession and the public to accept the nurse-midwife. During the early 1970s, some nurse-midwives began calling for enabling legislation which would separate nurse-midwifery from medicine and nursing. One nurse-midwife argued that 'in resurrecting the midwife, it was necessary to create the midwife from the nursing discipline which was held in the highest esteem . . . [but] as with every birthing process, it is time now to cut the umbilical cord.'

The controversy over whether nurse-midwifery should be separated from the nursing profession continues to this day, splitting the membership of the ACNM on this issue. Those who wish to stay within nursing argue that creating an independent midwifery profession would represent a greater challenge to the medical profession and that it would be disloyal to the profession of nursing. The nurse-midwives who do not want to be regulated within the nursing profession maintain that nursing is a separate profession, one based on the care of sick people, and, as such, has little to do with midwifery. They feel that loyalty to the nursing profession is misplaced and tends to keep nurse-midwives under the thumb of the medical profession. The anti-nursing faction within the ACNM wants to be free of the current stricture that requires written evidence of collaboration with a qualified physician before a nurse-midwife can practice. This limitation has kept many nurse-midwives from practicing, since there are many parts of the country in which a physician willing to enter into a written agreement with a nurse-midwife cannot be found.

WOMEN BEGIN TO SPEAK OUT

The first half of the century was an era in which women were generally so submissive that there was almost no expression from them regarding their birth experiences. Things began to change in 1958 with an avalanche of letters sent to a national women's magazine (*Ladies' Home Journal*) following a single letter from a registered nurse who dared not sign her name for fear of reprisal. Her letter complained about the cruelty she had witnessed on maternity wards, and the *Journal* invited readers to comment. Letters from mothers all over the country were published, and the nurse's charges were corroborated. Readers complained about being strapped hand and foot on delivery tables and being left for hours. Many others charged that their legs were held together by nurses to hold back the birth until the doctor arrived, a practice that sometimes caused brain damage in the babies. The *Journal* finished the year by publishing a list of recommendations for reform.[7]

It was during the late 1950s and early 1960s that the first childbirth education organizations were formed: the International Childbirth Education Association and the American Society for Psychoprophylaxis in Childbirth. A new philosophy of family-centered maternity care and consumer rights in health care was born. Women in certain parts of the country were able for the first time to attend classes in childbirth preparation and to have the support of an organization behind them when they requested permission for their husbands to be with them during labor and delivery in hospitals.

A boost to the budding childbirth reform movement came with a startlingly new phenomenon that began in the mid-1960s in northern California. The *Zeitgeist* of the 1960s was already characterized by the widespread questioning of authority by the generation that was coming of age. Hundreds of thousands of young people saw the need to take a radical departure from an unquestioning acceptance of ideas and edicts that came from what they called the Establishment. The counter-culture's strong belief in the natural order of things led to a growing perception among young people that the birth process should not necessarily require the presence of thousands of dollars of technological equipment in order to come to a safe and satisfactory conclusion. The thalidomide tragedy in Europe reinforced many women's growing suspicions that obstetricians were too often careless with and ignorant about women's bodies. More than 5,000 children with missing extremities and other major abnormalities were born in Britain, Japan, West Germany, Scandinavia, Italy, Argentina, Brazil and other nations. Damages paid to families of victims reached approximately $100 million, while not all families were compensated.[8] Hundreds of young women refused to submit to maternity care as provided to women within the mainstream of society. Instead of going to the hospital when labor began, they stayed at home to give birth.

The women who began serving as birth attendants at home births were usually college-educated, but not within medical disciplines. Often these women had had negative experiences of their own while giving birth in hospitals and had a sense of mission about protecting their friends from uncompassionate treatment and unnecessary intervention within hospitals. I remember well the excitement I felt when, newly arrived in California, I talked to a woman who had had a home birth. Like me, she had had her first baby in a hospital in 1966. She had also had a routine forceps delivery with caudal anesthesia. What got to me was the way she described her home birth, which had been attended by a close friend who was an obstetrical nurse. This time she had no forced anesthesia, no razor nicks from a close and fast shave, and no episiotomy or tear. After the baby was born, she said, she looked to the window and saw the neighbor's cows looking in. They had walked a quarter of a mile up the road to look in that window. From that moment on, I knew that I would give birth again and that it wouldn't be in a hospital.

News of home births spread like wildfire, and birth practices within hospitals in northern California quickly began to shift in order to accommodate the new kind of assertive woman, one who might have a temper tantrum in a labor room if her partner was not permitted to be with her. Within a short time, husbands, friends, relatives, and even the baby's siblings were allowed to be present during labor and delivery, and hospital maternity rooms were decorated to seem more 'home-like', a way of soothing the sensibilities of this new generation of better-informed mothers.

Meanwhile, the new midwives set about learning the skills they would need to provide safe prenatal care for the women whose births they would attend. Some were taught basic skills, such as dilation checking, taking blood pressures, charting, urine checking, and monitoring foetal heart tones, by helpful nurses or, more rarely, by nurse-midwives. Others, myself included, learned these skills from physicians who believed that they had an ethical duty to support midwives. Many of the midwives formed study groups so they could share knowledge and give one another support.

Interestingly, women interested in childbirth began serving as attendants in different parts of the country, unaware of one another, an illustration of how much this new kind of midwifery was an expression of the *Zeitgeist*. For all some of us knew, we were the only kind of midwives in the country; I, for instance, was not aware of the existence of nurse-midwives until I had already begun attending births on my own. Because I lived in a southeastern state, I did know that traditional midwives still provided maternity services primarily for black women in rural areas of other southeastern states.

The effect of a few hundred home births was amplified greatly when some of the new midwives and other childbirth activists began to publish books about childbirth, often contrasting the hospital mode of birth with home birth. Raven Lang's *Birth Book* (1972),[9] my *Spiritual Midwifery* (1975),[10] Lester Hazell's *Commonsense Childbirth* (1976),[11] and Rahima Baldwin's *Special Delivery* (1979)[12] helped to fuel the movement, as did books by activists such as Suzanne Arms with *Immaculate Deception* (1975),[13] the Boston Women's Health Book Collective's *Our Bodies, Our Selves* (1976),[14] and Doris Haire's influential pamphlet, *The Cultural Warping of Childbirth* (1972).[15] Associations of midwives formed, as did more organizations providing information and instruction about childbirth: how to get through labor, how to coach someone else through labor, how to avoid unnecessary episiotomies, and how to avoid the pitfalls of laboring in an unsupportive atmosphere within a hospital. A new type of public interest organization came into being in the 1980s: the group whose prime purpose was to reverse rapid increase in the national caesarean rate. Still another innovation, the out of hospital birth center, began to provide a new option for some mothers who wanted to give birth in a less medicalized atmosphere. By the middle of the 1980s, there were approximately 120 birth centers scattered throughout the country, most of them providing midwifery care to middle-income mothers.

Since the 1970s, despite the legal obstacles and the lack of officially approved educational programs, a few thousand American women have become midwives trained to provide prenatal and home birth service. Some work legally; others do not. Every one of the fifty American states has a different law regarding what is called 'direct-entry' midwifery, the stream of midwifery educaton that does not have nursing as a pre-requisite.* Several states have licensing mechanisms for direct-entry midwives, while in others, the only midwives who can legally work are nurse-midwives. Some people in every state, regardless of the legality of midwifery, continue to prefer the home birth option, and these people only rarely are able to enjoy the service of a nurse-midwife. Only a handful of nurse-midwives are able to provide domiciliary service, because almost no physicians can be found who will enter into a written agreement with any midwife to provide care for home births.

Because there is no national health service in the United States and one's right to maternity care is not assured, there exists a vacuum of care in many areas. This vacuum is often filled by direct-entry midwives. With very few exceptions, I would say that these women are competent, as well as conscientious. They take care of the women who do not have access to nurse-midwives in birth centers or hospitals, the women who are frightened of the high intervention rates in their local hospitals, the women who have no insurance coverage and who do not want to have their care begin in the emergency room of their local hospital once labor begins. The truth is that while paying for maternity care in the United States, whether through insurance or directly, does not guarantee good maternity care, not being able to pay for maternity care almost certainly guarantees the kind of poor care that is caused by understaffing, bad attitudes on the part of care providers, and an overdependence upon technology.

With only 3,000 or so nurse-midwives in a country of 250 million people, it is easy to see why so many direct-entry midwives have responded to the calls of women for their kind of care. Most nurse-midwives work in urban areas, and even then there are so few of them that relatively few American women have access to a nurse-midwife.

Criminal charges have been brought against a number of direct-entry midwives in California since 1974. There have been a few such charges in other states. Despite these arrests, thousands

* Ina May Gaskin here uses the term 'direct-entry' to mean 'empirical', 'lay' or 'independent'.

of midwives throughout the country continue to attend home births. In almost every instance of indictment or disciplinary action against a midwife, the midwives were brought to the attention of authorities by physicians or other medical personnel, not by the affected client.

Unlike the midwives of the early twentieth century, modern-day midwives have shown considerable energy in joining together to establish newsletters, to formulate competency standards in midwifery, and to lobby for midwifery legislation. Direct-entry midwifery has been legalized in several states, but not all midwives would agree that the results of legalization have been positive. In Florida, for instance, after years of strenuous lobbying, the Florida Midwives Association convinced the state legislature to pass a law providing for the education of direct-entry midwives and legalizing them. Two years later, after the midwives themselves had established two schools of direct-entry midwifery, the state legislature, under extreme pressure from the physicians' lobby, threw out the law legalizing direct-entry midwifery. Only the relatively small number of women who had been able to obtain their midwifery education during the two-year period of legalization could then be licenced. The door was closed.

Some of the state laws, again, because of medical pressure during the lawmaking process, contain regulations prohibiting the use of drugs used for treating hemorrhage after childbirth. Midwives who work under these conditions are forced to lie, for fear of losing their licences, or to jeopardize the safety of mothers by doing without drugs which most consider to be a necessary part of the domiciliary midwife's supplies. Other licenced midwives complain that they are, in effect, punished for transferring women who develop complications during labor to the hospital, because of the surveillance and harassment of regulatory agencies regarding these cases.

The American College of Nurse Midwives, caught between the home birth movement and the gatekeepers of American birth, the American College of Obstetricians and Gynecologists (ACOG), has plotted a careful course. The ACNM's position statement of 1973, which endorsed only 'hospital or officially approved maternity home as the site for childbirth,' was replaced by a 1980 pronouncement on 'practice settings,' which did include the home as an acceptable place for childbirth attended by a nurse-midwife.

The ACOG, on the other hand, has let stand its 1980 barrage of press releases to the national media. The ACOG statement referred to home birth as 'child abuse,' based upon information purported to have been gathered from '48 state departments of health' that supposedly proved that infant death in home births was two to five times greater than in hospital birth. The national media, as a general rule, tend to accept the pronouncements of any professional medical organization without question, and the ACOG statement on home birth was no exception. Few people outside the home birth movement were aware that the charge was highly questionable. Only eleven departments of health even had data available on infant mortality, and the category of out-of-hospital births in all of them included planned and unplanned deliveries (the births that occur on freeways, in taxis, elevators, cars, and other accidental places).

In 1982, a new organization, the Midwives Alliance of North America (MANA) was formed to unite midwives from all educational streams and to promote a strong vision of midwifery as an independent, self-regulating profession that recognizes multiple education routes to midwifery.

The Children's Defense Fund, a public interest organization, in a report released in early 1987, states that the United States has slipped to last place among twenty industrialized nations in reducing overall infant death rates. 'A key major factor that distinguishes the United States from countries that have reduced infant mortality rates more rapidly is the provision of maternity services,' the report said. 'Of all industrialized countries, the United States stands alone in its failure to assure pregnant women access to prenatal care and delivery services through either a public health service or universal health insurance.'

The rapidly increasing rate of teenage pregnancy in the United States is one of the factors aggravating an already bad situation. Teen mothers often do not know, or are afraid to admit, that they are pregnant, so that many go through pregnancies without any prenatal care. A growing number have what have been labelled by the media as 'toilet births,' that is, births which take place in toilets at schools or fast food restaurants. The babies are abandoned and are discovered by other schoolgirls or janitors. There were five such births reported during 1986 in Nashville, Tennessee.

Another peculiarly American phenomenon regarding child-birth is a relatively new practice called 'patient dumping.' Formerly, each state had a number of hospitals which would provide free maternity care to low-income, uninsured mothers. The number of hospitals willing to provide care to people unable to pay has decreased dramatically during the 1980s, with the rise of corporate medicine, advertising on billboards, television, and print media to attract patients, and business people determining hospital policies. Many hospitals which used to accept a certain percentage of laboring women who were uninsured or unable to pay for their care at entry to the hospital are no longer accepting these women. Instead, they are often sent to public hospitals, at a time when public hospitals are financially hard-pressed to provide free care.

During the late 1970s, Alabama, one of the states with a high infant mortality rate, began de-licencing the midwives who had served the rural black population, not because the midwives were incompetent or guilty of bad practice, but because federal money, through the Medicaid program, would pay for hospital births for rural low-income mothers. The midwives had no right of appeal or political voice, so by 1980 it was no longer legal for a midwife to attend a birth in a state where more than 200 midwives had been attending births just ten years earlier. No one in the state legislature or the state health department had foreseen that federal money would become scarce very soon after the midwives were prohibited from attending births. Meanwhile many mothers who had once been entitled to maternity benefits soon found that they were no longer eligible for free care. The midwives tried to resolve this problem by being present at births and coaching husbands to catch the babies. When health department authorities became aware of this practice, husbands were told that they, too, could be prosecuted for delivering their babies. The *Huntsville Times* printed a series of articles in 1984 about how overburdened the public hospitals were with providing indigent care and that some were going to have to close their doors to patients unable to pay. I am told by some of the de-licenced midwives that many women are now forced to give birth with no trained attendant at all. No effective measures have yet been instituted to remedy this situation.

The medical profession, far from having any answers to the

problems of lack of access to maternity care and the increase in teenage pregnancy, concentrates its attention primarily on two areas: high-tech solutions to the problems of infertility and the malpractice insurance issue. Because the American system lacks any mechanism for public accountability, and because there is no insurance to benefit families with birth-injured babies, people have come to see a lawsuit as their only way to defend themselves against bad practice or, in some cases, to acquire enough money to pay major medical bills. Courts have made large awards to parents who have brought malpractice suits against obstetricians in recent years, and insurance companies have responded by raising premium rates for malpractice insurance for obstetricians. Physicians' groups are pressuring state legislatures to pass laws placing ceilings on malpractice awards. It is too early to assess how successful such legislative attempts will be. Meanwhile, many obstetricians have given up their obstetrical practices and have concentrated instead on gynecology.

Obstetricians have another problem: that of oversupply and maldistribution. One federal commission recently estimated that the United States has at least 10,000 too many obstetricians, an estimate that is not hard to believe when we consider that the Office of Technology Assessment and Scientific Manpower Commission projects that the United States will have a surplus of 190,000 physicians (of all categories) by 1990. To compound the oversupply problem, obstetricians mostly prefer to live in urban areas, which leaves rural and small town areas chronically underserved.

Whether or not the American public will choose to promote legislation to remove legal barriers to midwifery, to limit the number of physicians, including obstetricians, or to create any incentives for better distribution remains to be seen. Until then, it is likely that midwives will continue to face intense competition from the medical profession in their efforts to promote midwifery as a profession. At the same time, American women's desire for midwifery care seems to be growing.

It is difficult to see how midwifery can become established as a strong and independent profession in the United States unless midwives are able to enter into coalitions with organizations with similar aims. Before midwives can take really effective steps in this direction, it is likely that midwives from the different streams of American midwifery will have to overcome their mutual suspicions of one another and to develop a real sense of solidarity among themselves. The founding of the Midwives Alliance of North America represents the first baby steps in this direction. Now the task is to learn to walk.

NOTES

1 De Tocqueville, Alexis, *Democracy in America*, edited and abridged by Richard Heffner, New American Library, 1963.

2 Wertz, Richard W. and Wertz, Dorothy C., *Lying-In: A History of Childbirth in America*, Schocken Books, 1979.

3 DeLee, Joseph B., 'The prophylactic forceps operation,' paper presented at the Forty-fifth Annual Meeting of the American Gynecological Society, Chicago, 24–26 May 1920.

4 Axelsen, Diana E., 'Women as victims of medical experimentation,' *Sage: A Scholarly Journal on Black Women*, vol. 2, no. 2, Fall, 1985.

5 Litoff, Judy Barrett, *American Midwives: 1860 to the Present*, Greenwood Press, 1978.

6 Breckinridge, Mary, *Wide Neighborhoods*, University Press of Kentucky, 1981.

7 Waldorf, Mary and Edwards, Margot, *Reclaiming Birth*, Crossing Press, 1984.

8 'Help for the helpers,' *Time*, 30 April 1973.

9 Lang, Raven, *Birth Book*, Genesis, 1972.

10 Gaskin, Ina May, *Spiritual Midwifery*, revised edn, Book Publishing Co., 1978.

11 Hazell, Lester, *Commonsense Childbirth*, Berkley Press, 1976.

12 Baldwin, Rahima, *Special Delivery*, Les Femmes, 1977.

13 Arms, Suzanne, *Immaculate Deception*, Houghton Mifflin, 1975.

14 Boston Women's Health Book Collective, *Our Bodies, Ourselves*, Simon & Schuster, 1976.

15 Haire, Doris B., *The Cultural Warping of Childbirth*, International Childbirth Education Association, 1972.

DIRECT-ENTRY MIDWIFERY IN THE USA

JO ANNE MYERS-CIECKO

Eleven years ago, in 1976, I had my first baby at home in Seattle, Washington, with the loving support of family and friends and the assistance of two young midwives. Like most American women giving birth, I was not particularly well-informed. However, unlike my contemporaries, I had sought out mid-wifery care when it was suggested by my friends.

I was not completely sure of my decision to have the baby at home, so I also visited an obstetrician several times in early pregnancy. I abandoned that effort when it became clear that his prenatal care routine was strictly limited to the most minimal clinical assessment and that he seemed to lack any genuine interest in me as a whole person, allowing no time for my questions and concerns about my pregnancy and birth. My midwives, in contrast, were part of a feminist women's health collective, clearly committed to providing an alternative to standard medical care. Prenatal visits were an opportunity for long conversations about how I was feeling, how my work was going, what my plans were for the rest of the pregnancy and more. Still, a little voice inside kept nagging at me about the lack of medical sanction for the midwives' practice and the safety of home birth.

It was not until very near the end of my pregnancy that I realized it was really *me* that was going to have the baby. No amount of wishful thinking or placing responsibility on a physi-cian or midwife was going to change the fact that the baby was inside me and that I would have a role in its birth. I wanted an environment in which I would feel the most empowered to labor and give birth. The hospital represented a tantalizing temptation to believe that I could give the responsibility over to someone else. But when I really thought about the implications of routine anesthesia, episiotomy or caesarean section, I saw that those would still have an impact on my body and my baby. So I made peace with the decision to stay at home and I found the incredible strength I needed from my friends and the confidence I needed under the watchful eyes and hands of my midwives.

Little did I realize that my own personal experience was one small part of a major new phase in the development of the midwifery profession in the United States; that events in Washington State over the next ten years would be part of a national struggle to define, promote and legitimize midwifery; or that the midwives who attended me that night would one day themselves come to represent the diversity of midwifery training, practice, and philosophy that now exists in the US. One of those midwives went on to pursue education in nursing and nurse-midwifery, eventually working as a certified nurse-midwife in a busy urban hospital, serving a low-income, often high-risk clientele. The other midwife has continued her independent home birth practice and has been a major force in the creation of a direct-entry midwifery school accredited by the State of Washington, and often cited as an example of a new brand of professional midwifery in North America.

Midwives in the US are the primary attendants at less than 5 per cent of all births.[1] Although this percentage has risen steadily for the last ten years, most people are only vaguely aware of midwives. They don't know that midwifery has an essentially different orientation to childbearing than medicine or that today's modern midwives provide complex, high-quality care. They certainly don't appreciate the legal or professional distinctions made between midwives from various educational backgrounds or legal categories.

Public demand for the services of midwives and acceptance by other health care professionals has been confounded by the particular history of midwifery and childbirth in the United States. The number of midwives declined steadily from the turn of this century in direct relation to the consolidation of power among physicians and the medicalization of childbirth. A resurgence in the practice of midwifery began in the 1970s with increased concern over the quality and cost of obstetric care.

Faced with many obstacles to their practice and a general lack of support, midwives have been divided among themselves as to how the profession might be strengthened.

Today there are approximately 2,300 certified nurse-midwives (CNMs) in the US.[2] CNMs are registered nurses (graduates of nursing programs of two, three or four years' duration) who have completed additional training in midwifery. They must complete a certificate, master's degree, or doctoral prgram accredited by the American College of Nurse-Midwives (ACNM) and pass a national certification examination administered by the ACNM. While the ACNM has established guidelines for the functions, standards and qualification of certified nurse-midwives, their practice is actually regulated at the state level like that of all other health professionals. In most states, nurse-midwifery practice is overseen by the State Board of Nursing. Regulations concerning the level of education, actual scope of practice, prescriptive authority, relationships with physicians, and even the site of practice vary considerably from state to state.[3]

State regulations concerning the practice of midwifery outside of nursing are even more diverse, ranging from clear prohibition to recognition of lay midwives who have completed apprenticeships to licensure for graduates of direct-entry midwifery schools.[4] Terminology describing the training and legal and professional status of midwives is equally confusing. 'Lay,' 'direct-entry' and 'independent' are commonly used interchangeably to describe the midwife who is not a certified nurse-midwife. Lacking nationally established definitions and in the face of a general absence of understanding by other professionals, it is not surprising that this confusion persists. For the purposes of this discussion, I will use the term 'direct-entry' broadly to include midwives who have completed a prescribed course of training that meets the requirements for state licensing or state midwifery association certification and who are not CNMs. This will arbitrarily exclude some midwives who do not have access to legal or professional recognition but who may be well qualified to practice midwifery. At the same time, it will include some midwives who would not qualify as direct-entry if we were to use the term strictly as it was borrowed from midwifery in Great Britain and Europe. One can estimate, using this definition, that there are several hundred direct-entry midwives in the country and perhaps several thousand other midwives.

How is it that midwifery came to be so misunderstood by the general public and other health professionals? Why is there such a lack of conformity regarding midwifery training and standing and how has that contributed to the lack of communication, trust and unity of purpose among midwives? How have circumstances changed in the last ten to twenty years to create new hope that the midwife may eventually come to be seen as the appropriate caregiver for most childbearing women?

I believe that women in the 1960s, 1970s and 1980s have quite unconsciously inherited a legacy of bias against midwifery and an all-pervasive belief that childbirth is a pathological state. Our grandmothers were all too aware of the risks associated with childbearing at the turn of the century. Although vital data was only beginning to be collected and figures are sketchy, it appears that the maternal mortality rate was extremely high, perhaps as much as one maternal death for every 154 babies born alive.[5] While we now understand that most of these deaths could have been prevented with improved economic conditions, reduced birth rates, and better control of infections, many physicians at the time blamed the problem on midwives. Professional journals and the popular press encouraged debate on the 'midwife problem' among these physicians and public health officials.

At the same time, our grandmothers were interested in making birth not only safer but also less painful. They were among early feminists who, in a burst of enthusiasm for reducing the risks and pains of childbirth, organized a national movement to demand the use of 'twilight sleep' or anesthesia in birth. Unfortunately their efforts backfired when it turned out that hospitalization and the medicalization of birth, in fact, removed much of the strength women had derived from their own surroundings, and the support of friends and family.[6]

By the time our mothers were having babies, most births occurred in hospitals and very few women experienced birth as a normal event. Many now have only nightmarish recollections of being alone among strangers during labor, of drugged births, and separation from the baby and other family following childbirth.[7] Breastfeeding was not encouraged and very little was known about its benefits to mother and infant. Consequently, few of us grow up with information provided by our mothers that would prepare us for childbearing as a normal physiological process or a family-centered cultural event.

In the last ten years obstetric technology has become ever more sophisticated, with more tests and interventions than ever.[8] Despite pressure from women and their families to humanize the birth experience, control over the circumstances and course of birth remains firmly in the hands of the medical profession. There have been a few concessions such as allowing fathers to participate in births and discarding routine procedures like enemas and pubic shaves in most communities. However, women's underlying fears of the pain and potential danger of childbirth remains.

Most women choose standard medical practices which give the appearance of guaranteeing that childbirth can be made painless and entirely safe. Now physicians and the public alike are suffering from the effects of such underlying assumptions. Steeply rising malpractice insurance premiums and the fear of lawsuits are causing physicians to practice ever more defensively. Routine prenatal diagnostic ultrasound and continued high rates of caesarean section are but two examples of defensive medical practices that persist contrary to the advice of national experts.

Because health care is a commodity for sale in the US, there are also certain economic pressures brought to bear on obstetrics. Hospitals must maintain the latest in sophisticated equipment to attract both physicians and patients. There is generally a good return on their investments in maternity services where there is high utilization of expensive equipment and procedures and a rapid turnover of patients.[9] At the same time, to compete in the marketplace where consumers are looking for more options in their birthing experiences, hospitals use billboards and newspaper advertisements to promote their 'family-centered care.' Natural childbirth and anesthesia are portrayed as if they were entrées on a buffet table of birthing options. A woman touring the hospital near the end of her pregnancy will be told that episiotomies are no longer routine. Yet she will most likely have an episiotomy because her physician is neither comfortable with nor skilled in managing births over an intact perineum. She will, of course, be told that it was necessary to avoid a more painful or difficult-to-repair laceration.

Under the best conditions, most women will feel that they had some power to plan and choose among alternatives for their birth experience. At the same time, they will likely have been 'rescued' from pain and/or danger by the nursing and medical staff. It's no small wonder that the message from midwifery advocates characterizing birth as a natural and joyful event is received skeptically by the general population (not to mention other health care professionals).

These modern perceptions of childbearing do not, however, completely explain the biases against midwives. For that, we must go back to the beginning of the twentieth century for a closer look at the history of midwifery in the United States.[10]

It is reported that midwives delivered approximately one-half of the babies born in the United States in 1910. The two largest groups of midwives at the time were professional midwives trained in Europe and lay midwives called into service by friends and neighbors. There was generally no licensure or official recognition afforded these midwives, nor were they organized professionally. The few schools of midwifery that existed in the US were short-lived, independent schools or programs initiated by local public health officials in an attempt to improve local maternal child health outcomes. Bellevue School for Midwives in New York City was probably the most notable example of a municipally sponsored program, founded in 1911 and surviving until 1935 when a lack of students forced its closure.

Physicians, in contrast, had been organizing for several decades under the auspices of the American Medical Association. Licensing requirements were becoming more stringent. There was pressure to upgrade medical education. Most physicians were not well-trained according to the Flexner Report of 1910, which criticized the lack of clinical training in medical schools. Other studies done in the first quarter of the century attributed many poor outcomes to poor medical practices that led to otherwise preventable problems such as puerperal fever and birth injuries. Some prominent physicians responded to these criticisms by attacking the midwives. Their slanderous campaign eventually proved quite effective, as midwives and the public health officials who came to their defense were vulnerable to the organized power of the physicians.

The professional midwives were for the most part immigrants

who had trained in Europe or Asia and who served the women of their own ethnic communities. They often did not speak English and were subject to the same racist and ethnic prejudices felt by all immigrants. They did not cross their racial or ethnic boundaries to join forces, establish professional organizations, develop schools, influence health policy, or resist the pressures at work to usurp midwifery's role in the provision of maternity care. Their numbers dwindled as the midwives aged, the supply of new immigrants ended with changing immigration laws, and second-generation women aspired to the services offered to upper- and middle-class women.[11]

Lay midwives were mainly black women ('granny midwives') in impoverished rural areas of the south, Native American women on the Indian reservations, Chicana women in Texas and the southwest ('*parteras*'), and women in the widely scattered and isolated mining, grazing or homesteading communities west of the Mississippi River. The percentage of births attended by these midwives, particularly in the southern and southwestern states, did not drop off as rapidly as it did for the immigrant midwives. In 1948 it was estimated that there were over 20,000 practicing lay midwives in the US. By 1976, the estimated total was 1,800, almost half of whom were located in Texas. In 1940, midwife deliveries among nonwhites were still at 49 per cent while the corresponding figure for whites was 3.5 per cent. In the southern state of Mississippi, midwives still attended 7.7 per cent of all births in 1970 and 15.7 per cent among nonwhites.[12] Many states provided legal sanction for the practices of these midwives whose activities were often supervised by local public health officials. Their contribution to the provision of maternity care to otherwise underserved populations – the rural, the poor, and the racial minorities – was significant.[13]

The concept of nurse-midwifery first entered discussions concerning midwifery in the 1910s, but as we have seen in Ina May Gaskin's chapter, the first successful model for nurse-midwifery practice was Mary Breckenridge's Frontier Nursing Service. The clinical service and the school received national recognition for significantly improving the maternal and child health of this impoverished region and demonstrating the effectiveness of nurse-midwifery practice.

In the meantime, the Maternity Center Association had been

founded in New York City in 1918 to combat the city's high maternal and infant mortality rates through provision of prenatal care, education, and care for women delivering in their homes. In 1923, the MCA made an agreement with Bellevue School for Midwives to provide instruction in midwifery to the MCA's nurses, but the plan was rejected by the city commissioner of welfare. It was not until 1934 that the MCA began its own midwifery training program. MCA graduates went on to work in many other states, supervising granny midwives in the south, and establishing nurse-midwifery schools in Alabama and New Mexico.

Yet despite the impressive records of the Frontier Nursing Service and the Maternity Center Association, the nurse-midwifery concept did not flourish. The dramatic decline in midwife-attended births in the first quarter of the century was not reversed and, in fact, continued for another fifty years into the 1970s.

The first efforts to control and improve the quality of nurse-midwifery education were organized through the Nurse-Midwifery Section of the National Organization for Public Health Nursing.[14] In the early 1950s, the major nursing organizations regrouped and the National League for Nursing assumed the activities of the National Organization of Public Health Nursing. There was no longer a separate section provided for nurse-midwives. Without support from the national nursing organization and still wanting to establish standards for nurse-midwifery education as well as a means for promoting the profession, the nurse-midwives founded the American College of Nurse-Midwives in 1955.

Ten years later, a study conducted by the Children's Bureau of the US Department of Health, Education and Welfare reported that there were approximately 750 graduates of American nurse-midwifery schools, though fewer than forty were actually engaged in the practice of nurse-midwifery or were providing nurse-midwifery education.[15] The others were teaching in maternal-child health nursing, were obstetric nurse supervisors, staff nurses, supervisors of public health nurses or local midwives, were engaged in research or parent education, or were pursuing other baccalaureate education.

Several demonstration projects had been established to

examine the benefits of utilizing nurse-midwives and showed good results. In 1960–63, two nurse-midwives were employed in a pilot project in a poor farming community in California. They managed the care, including deliveries, of the majority of patients. Prematurity and neonatal deaths were significantly reduced during this period and rose again dramatically when the demonstration project was discontinued.[16]

In 1968 The Macy Foundation sponsored a conference on 'The Midwife in the United States' which included several speakers critical of US infant mortality figures, the discrepancy in care provided to nonwhite women, and the overcrowded conditions of maternity units in urban ghettos.[17] It was suggested that nurse-midwives offered a solution to these problems. One example cited the Columbia University's School of Nursing Graduate Program in Maternity Nursing which had organized a nurse-midwife service at Harlem Hospital, a site typical of many overcrowded, neglected and understaffed maternity units in New York City. The nurse-midwife staff was able to make a significant improvement in the quality of care under difficult conditions and were highly respected for their dedication to patients and family-centered care.

At this time there were about ten nurse-midwifery schools offering either certificates or graduate degrees. All but the Frontier Nursing Service were university-based or affiliated. Standards for training and clinical practice were influenced by this proximity to major medical and nursing schools. During the 1950s and 1960s, reports emphasized that nurse-midwives were to be seen as members of the perinatal health care team, assistants to the physician, functioning only in medical centers and as employees of institutions. The nurse-midwife was not generally envisioned as a private practitioner nor was it anticipated that she would ever return to domiciliary service.

There was ongoing discussion about the midwife's relationship to nursing. The Macy Conference Report includes themes that sound strikingly familiar twenty years later. Should nursing regulatory bodies have authority over midwifery practice? Should midwifery be considered a clinical nursing specialty? What are the benefits and drawbacks to this association between nursing and midwifery?

By the late 1960s, the American College of Nurse-Midwives

had developed a process for accrediting educational programs and voluntary accreditation was underway by 1970. A committee had been charged with developing a national certification examination for nurse-midwives. The ACNM membership voted in 1971 to require a national examination as the basis for certification and it was first offered that year.

During the period from 1940 to 1970, as Ina May Gaskin has shown, a movement to reform childbirth emerged.[18] Women, reacting to the heavy use of anesthesia in labor, advocated the more 'natural childbirth' orientation of physicians like Dr Grantly Dick-Read and Dr Ferdinand Lamaze. The La Lèche League was founded by a group of mothers in Chicago in 1956 to encourage the nearly lost art of breastfeeding. The International Childbirth Education Association, a federation of parent groups, was founded in 1960 affirming a belief in family-centered birth, a conviction that birth belongs to the parents and not the hospital, and a philosophy of consumer rights in health care.

Very gradually there were changes made in the routines of maternity care, including organization of childbirth education classes, hospital policy reforms such as allowing the father into the labor room, a change from general anasthesia to the spinal block, and so on. However, despite these hard-won concessions to consumer demand, the medical model of birth (pathology and medical control) remained secure. 'Natural childbirth' had many meanings and frequently included episiotomy, outlet forceps, Demerol, and epidural anesthesia. Women, wanting to believe that they had been successful in having a natural birth, were encouraged to accept these routine interventions as components of a natural birth by physicians who believed that medical personnel should have control over the birth experience.

In the 1960s and 1970s, the US experienced tremendous social upheaval. The Cold War, the civil rights movement, the War on Poverty, the anti-war and feminist movements all had an impact on maternal-child health policies, midwifery practice, and women's view of themselves.

A physician shortage was predicted in the early 1960s following a period when public priorities were committed to training scientists and engineers to develop military and space technology for the Cold War. The Kennedy Administration responded to these predictions with increased funding for medical education.

Thus began a trend of medical school expansion that leaves us in the 1980s with gloomy predictions of a physician glut.[19]

The civil rights movement and War on Poverty, meanwhile, were setting changes in motion that would lead to the elimination of the granny midwives in the south. Demands for desegregation of medical facilities and equal access to medical care were to lead to a steep decline in midwifery practice. Despite several decades of official sanction through state licencing and training and supervision provided by public health officials, these midwives became *personae non gratae*. Blacks themselves, with a desire to improve their status and well-being, aspired to the same privileges enjoyed by white families and rejected the old-style midwives. It is interesting to note that these policies worked in favor of eliminating the midwives rather than providing incentives for the development of their professional status. There does not appear to have been any discussion during this time of providing money for midwifery education.

With the Johnson Administration's declaration of a 'War on Poverty' and the establishment of the national system of medical benefits for impoverished families, new money became available for the provision of health care and the reimbursement of mainstream providers, namely physicians. This further encouraged the transfer of care to physicians.

The anti-war movement and the civil rights movement fostered a renewed interest, particularly among young people, in the democratic traditions of the United States. As in the Jacksonian period of the first half of the nineteenth century, self-help movements, alternative health care models, and a focus on the individual's role in their own health care were common features of dissident communities' ideals.

These, in turn, created a new feminist movement among women frustrated with male power and political models. They further developed the self-help and alternative models in philosophical and practical works such as the Boston Women's Health Book Collective's landmark *Our Bodies, Our Selves*.[20] Study groups and women's clinics encouraged women to learn about their bodies and to take more responsibility for their own health care. Unable to rely on the male medical model or mainstream physicians, many clinics were staffed by paraprofessionals.

While much of this effort focused on reproductive health issues such as contraception, sterilization and abortion rights, there were a few women across the country who turned their attention to the childbearing experience. With hospitals and physicians seemingly hopelessly mired down in their pathologic models of pregnancy and birth, these women strove to create an alternative which would empower the woman herself. Home births attended by these new midwives emerged as a new model for maternity care.[21]

There were also movements which had an orientation to the more spiritual aspect of birth and promoting alternative life-styles. Some of these people were moving back to the land or looking to develop alternatives to the unhealthy and materially wasteful lifestyles of mainstream American culture. It was quite natural for these women to turn to one another in childbirth, creating a new generation of midwives in the tradition of their ancestors.

Meanwhile, certified nurse-midwives saw themselves as pioneers in their own right, veterans of the battle to establish themselves professionally. In 1970, they were only just beginning to see the results of decades of groundwork, in expanded educational and work opportunities, and in growing legal and professional recognition. They had persisted in the face of seemingly insurmountable odds, determined to bring high-quality care to women in remote rural areas and urban ghettos. They had made inroads in some of the most powerful university teaching hospitals, working side by side with the residents who would one day practice obstetrics. They had established services in some of the worst public hospitals in the country and were managing to improve the quality of care for many women despite deplorable conditions.

They were advocates for improved quality of care and yet, when a new generation of childbearing women began to seek alternatives to standard medical care, nurse-midwives were often criticized for their unwillingness to leave or to condemn the practices of the institutions that they had worked so hard to infiltrate. It was true that the newer nurse-midwifery programs were established within universities and that clinical experience was generally limited to hospital births under close medical supervision. While more and more states were recognizing the practice of nurse-midwifery, there was considerable variation in the scope of practice allowed and the degree of physician supervision required. Some states required written agreements with a supervising physician and some restricted nurse-midwifery practice to in-hospital services. Given their historical struggle for survival, the many legal constraints, and their lack of training and experience in home births, it is not surprising that some nurse-midwives did not wholeheartedly embrace the birth reform and new midwifery movements that were pushing for more radical alternatives to medical care.

With little professional or governmental support, the various new midwives sought training and experience through whatever means were available or could be readily created. Study groups, correspondence courses, independent self-study, workshops and apprenticeships were the most common pathways to education outside of nurse-midwifery schools. Sympathetic nurse-midwives, physicians, and more experienced lay midwives all contributed to the creation of educational opportunities. Most of the new midwives were daughters of the middle class, well-educated, in their late twenties or thirties, independent and resourceful. They did not want to be nurses themselves, nor did they see the necessity of nursing as a prerequisite to midwifery practice. They saw an advantage in establishing midwifery as an independent profession able to define practice and set standards on its own terms in order to provide a meaningful alternative to the medical model of birth.

However, the struggle for legal recognition and public and professional acceptance of these new midwives was to prove no less complicated than it had been for nurse-midwifery. The legal status of midwifery varies considerably from one state to another. Whereas midwifery practice may be clearly illegal in one state, a neighboring state may only recognize graduates of direct-entry schools, and yet another may not regulate midwifery at all. Some midwives have been prosecuted for practicing medicine or midwifery illegally and have paid dearly for their convictions in personal and financial terms.

In states where there was existing favorable legislation, the struggle has taken other forms as efforts have been devoted to the creation of state-approved educational programs and the modernizing of old laws and regulations. Many state midwifery associations have emerged in response to the unique needs of the individual states. They perform a variety of functions, including political lobbying, educational activities, legal defense, and development of professional identity.

The tremendous diversity in the actual conditions experienced by midwives in different states, combined with regional variations in the history of nurse-midwifery and the second-class status of the old lay midwives, has made it extremely difficult to establish common goals for all midwives nationally.

In the late 1970s and early 1980s, there was discussion in the American College of Nurse-Midwives as to what relationship, if any, there should be between the ACNM and the new midwives.[22] By this time, there were several formally organized direct-entry training programs and an ever-increasing number of midwives legally practicing in states such as Washington, New Mexico and New Hampshire. Surveys were conducted, open forums held, and numerous articles written which addressed issues such as educational standards, professional qualifications, competency, and shared goals for maternal-child health.

Many CNMs argued in favor of increased avenues for communication and even for allowing other midwives access to an ACNM-sponsored national certification examination. For some this was primarily a practical response to the reality that other midwives were increasing in number and acceptance by consumers. For others it represented an opportunity to act on their own beliefs that midwifery should be a profession distinct from nursing. However, there was never sufficient agreement achieved within the ACNM to warrant a major change in policy concerning membership and qualifications for practicing midwifery.

Efforts to increase communication were frustrated by the lack of a comparable national organization. There were several groups, such as the National Association of Parents and Professionals for Safe Alternatives in Childbirth, which spoke out on behalf of midwifery. There were also groups such as the National Midwives Association which had not achieved a broad-based membership. In 1981, the President of the ACNM called a meeting of several midwives from around the country, in the hope of laying groundwork for a new organization which would represent the diversity of midwives and establish an official liaison with the ACNM.[23] The initial group, made up of lay, direct-entry, and certified nurse-midwives, was committed to expanding communication among all midwives, forming an identifiable professional organization, establishing educational guidelines and guidelines for basic competency and safety for practicing midwives. Eventually, this nucleus and the many other midwives that came forward in subsequent meetings founded the Midwives Alliance of North America (MANA).

In just a few years, MANA has contributed to increased and markedly improved communication among midwives in the United States.* It appears from the limited literature available on the subject and my own observations that all midwives would like to be acknowledged professionally and legally for their expertise in normal maternity care. There remain many obstacles to the achievement of that goal, not the least of which is a lack of clear consensus nationally as to how that recognition should be structured.

Many midwives are wary of legalization which might unduly limit their practice.[24] To the extent that the definition of normalcy and the accepted standards of care are determined by the medical/obstetric establishment, they may have reason for concern. There are ongoing examples of active prosecution, less overt persecution, and a general unwillingness to cooperate among physicians that encourage these feelings of caution. Likewise, there are concerns that the high cost of obtaining formal education that is typical of medicine, graduate nursing, and other professions, will be duplicated in the 'professionalization' of midwifery. There are many who maintain a strong commitment to apprenticeship, correspondence and other flexible avenues to training so as to encourage, rather than discourage, entry to the profession for those who would serve rural and low-income populations. There are also those who have had positive experiences with licensure; who enjoy greater public visibility and professional status; and who are making connections between midwifery and larger issues of public health policy.

* The organization and membership of MANA encompasses both the US and Canada. I refer here to the role of MANA in the development of midwifery in the US, but would like to remark that the dialogue and support between midwives from both countries has been an integral and significant part of MANA's evolution.

Despite these significant differences in experience and orientation, much has been accomplished by the members of MANA. Standards of practice have been adopted. A special section of MANA was created for those midwives who meet international standards and that section was granted membership of the International Confederation of Midwives (ICM). Considerable work has been done on developing the concepts of peer review, written protocols, professional ethics, data collection, research and certification. In 1986, the membership voted to establish an interim body to further develop a proposal for a national registry system.

Meanwhile, many state associations, not officially connected to MANA, have responded to conditions in their own states by creating state-level systems for credentialling midwives. State-level legislative efforts also go on independent of any nationally coordinated plan. While these activities reflect the reality of state regulation and the current level of national organization, we can foresee many complications in establishing reciprocity from state to state. The fact that nurse-midwives are generally regulated under a set of laws which is different again just adds to the complexity of establishing a clear and common identity for midwifery.

All of these issues – from standards of practice and regulation to appropriate educational models – are common themes in dicussions among nurse-midwives too. While there have been individual nurse-midwives who have been active in MANA, there has been very little official dialogue between MANA and the ACNM. This is likely to change as the ACNM comes to terms with the existence of another major midwifery organization in the US and as MANA is better able to articulate a position on the issues.

Some differences will probably persist between certified nurse-midwives and direct-entry midwives. The great majority of direct-entry midwives appear to be self-employed, private practitioners, doing home births and occasionally birth center deliveries. While the number of certified nurse-midwives working in this way has increased markedly in the last fifteen years, most are employed by hospitals, government agencies or private organizations, receive a salary, and are doing births in hospitals.[25]

Hospital-based practitioners are likely to do considerably more births per year and to serve different kinds of populations, including women with complications of pregnancy or labor whose care is provided by the midwife in collaboration with or under the supervision of a physician. Hospital-based practitioners also rely to varying degrees on other hospital staff, including nurses, aides, and technicians. They are not likely to sit at the side of one woman for the duration of her labor and may or may not have seen her prenatally as part of a group practice.

Midwives working in the home will generally see far fewer births per year and may not have the opportunity to participate in the care of women with complications requiring hospitalization. They are much more likely to attend to only one woman at a time in labor, having already seen her for complete prenatal care.

Neither of these models of midwifery care is an ideal and, of course, there are midwives, both nurse- and direct-entry, who are working somewhere in between these two ends of the spectrum. But what, then, is midwifery practice – how is it perceived by the public and by other professionals? What is the level of a midwife's responsibility? How do insurance companies and government agencies view the midwife's role and how should she be reimbursed for her services? As the provision of health care changes in the US, away from private independent practice and toward managed health care systems, how will midwives and their special contribution to the care of women fit into these new systems?

Midwives from diverse backgrounds, with experience and training along the entire spectrum of maternity services, have a great deal to learn from one another. Midwives in the United States, because of their unusually disrupted history, have the opportunity, as they work on the margins of mainstream obstetric care, to bring fresh insights to the definition of modern midwifery practice. They must be aware of their heritage – proud of what midwives have contributed to maternal-child health and well-informed as to the pitfalls of inadequate communication, organization, educational opportunities, and public support.

Ultimately midwives will flourish only as much as childbearing women and the society as a whole needs and values their services. There have been numerous state and federal investigations in recent years into such diverse issues as the use of electronic foetal ultrasound, reducing the incidence of low birth weight babies, the rising costs of health care, alternative birthing methods, and the malpractice crisis. Time and again, the recommendations of these groups have favored changes in medical practices and the increased utilization of midwives. More officials are recognizing that midwifery care can have a positive impact on the health and well-being of childbearing women.[26] Midwives provide care that supports the woman and her family, is culturally sensitive, emphasizes education, and reduces unnecessary interventions and our dependence on high-priced technology. As more women also recognize that birth can be a safe and more satisfying experience when supported by good midwifery care, midwives will be seen as an essential part of the health care system in the United States.

MIDWIVES IN WASHINGTON STATE

Washington State provides an interesting and somewhat unusual example of the situation for midwifery today in the United States. Growing unity among midwives and greater public visibility are hopeful indications of a brighter future for midwifery despite the challenges they face.

In 1972, the University of Washington School of Nursing sponsored a conference entitled 'Meeting the Consumer Challenge – Home Birth in the 1970s.'[27] Like many other states, there had been an increase in the reported number of home births in Washington. At the time it appears that there were no nurse-midwives in practice in Washington, although at least one conference participant was a nurse-midwife who taught in a local school of nursing. Apparently the home births were attended by a few physicians and some of the new generation of lay midwives, and questions about their practices did not arise.

By the mid-1970s, we know that there were many midwives practicing all over the state, including the highly visible feminist birth collective in Seattle that I had chosen to attend my first birth. In 1975 a Danish midwife, frustrated with the lack of opportunity to practice her profession, uncovered a 1917 Washington law that provided for the licensure of midwives. Her discovery came as a surprise to the state and to the midwives who had been practicing illegally. The Danish midwife was soon joined by a Chilean, an Australian, and several English-trained midwives as the first licensed midwives (LMs) recognized since the law had fallen into disuse in the 1930s. Although sanctioned by the state, their professional status was not generally understood or accepted by the medical community and their practices were restricted to attending home births. Many wound up back in labor and delivery units where they worked as nurses.

During this same period, several nurse-midwives joined forces to open the first free-standing birth centers in the state, becoming the first certified nurse-midwives to practice in Washington. Unlike the northeastern and southern United States where nurse-midwifery had a long history of attending low-income women and underserved communities, there was no such legacy in Washington. Likewise, there was no nurse-midwifery school or university/hospital-based nurse-midwifery service. This seems to have made it possible for a generation of relatively young, recently educated nurse-midwives to create a model of independent practice, sanctioned by the Board of Nursing. Soon a private group practice was also established within one hospital and a large health maintenance organization was preparing to try a pilot nurse-midwifery service.

Meanwhile, the State Department of Licensing was receiving more complaints about the illegally practicing lay midwives, and the medical association was lobbying the legislature to repeal the licensing law. Proponents of midwifery organized to defend the law and the feminist birth collective established a formal school in hopes of creating an avenue to licensure for practicing midwives. After several years of debate and negotiation, a revised law was passed in 1981 which incorporated international standards for midwifery education and practice.[28]

With more in common in their practices and their training than midwives in other states, the way was now open for the development of tentative relationships between certified nurse-midwives and licensed midwives. Nurse-midwives, while still wary of open association, were more accepting of these direct-entry midwives because of their identifiable educational preparation and legal status. The direct-entry midwives, likewise, sought the support of nurse-midwives who acted as consultants and instructors in the direct-entry school. Midwifery consumers and advocates also attempted to build bridges between the two professional groups by starting a newsletter which encouraged communication and supported the trials and tribulations of the two legally recognized kinds of midwives.

It took a crisis of major proportions, however, to forge a new professional organization representative of all midwives. A maternal death in a freestanding birth center and subsequent negative press coverage caused the midwives to come together in a series of meetings that culminated in the founding of the Midwives Association of Washington State (MAWS). In this organization, certified nurse-midwives and licensed midwives have worked together to identify standards for training and practice, to develop continuing education programs, and, most recently, to create a common peer review procedure for all midwives. This peer review program was also adopted by the local chapter of the American College of Nurse-Midwives, setting a precedent nationally for cooperation between organizations.

Since 1985, new problems have arisen for all midwives as a result of the general crisis in malpractice insurance. Both CNMs and LMs lost their group insurance coverage that year. However, many CNMs were covered by their employers and others were picked up on nursing policies while specific nurse-midwifery policies could be developed. The ACNM, fearing that they would be unable to find coverage, successfully lobbied Congress to revise the insurance laws, thereby enabling the ACNM to create its own self-insurance plan. This costly and all-consuming battle to obtain affordable insurance, a prerequisite to hospital privileges for private practitioners, has been the primary preoccupation of the ACNM for the last two years and seems to have discouraged any hope of formal links between CNMs and other midwives in much of the country. Licensed midwives, in contrast, have been without insurance altogether since 1985 and although most indicate that they would prefer insurance should it become available, they have been willing to continue their practices without it.[29]

Now all midwives in the state are increasingly feeling the loss or limitation of physician back-up as insurance companies and legal advisors put pressure on otherwise supportive physicians to limit consultation with other practitioners. This adds to already high stress levels for many midwives, including those whose hospital practices bring them into daily contact with hostile or defensive physicians and others whose options for securing consultation relationships are limited in rural communities and small towns. Stress, burn-out and turnover are common despite the personal rewards of working with birthing women.

Politically, the licensed midwives and certified nurse-midwives have joined forces to testify on one another's behalf as these and other obstacles to full practice are confronted. A licensed midwife applying for hospital privileges in a small community hospital in 1983, for instance, was supported in testimony by two certified nurse-midwives. Her application was eventually denied and it was not until 1986 that the first hospital in the state made it a policy to grant privileges to licensed midwives. One of the first with privileges happens to be in private practice with a certified nurse-midwife. When the Board of Nursing decided in 1986 to change the nursing regulations to require all nurse practitioners, including CNMs, to have a master's degree, licensed midwives protested alongside the certified nurse-midwives. When the midwifery licensure law was reviewed in 1985 and had to be repassed by the state legislature in 1986, CNMs joined LMs in raising money for a lobbyist to coordinate the legislative effort.

Licensed midwives and certified nurse-midwives in Washington State attended 4 per cent of all births in 1985, including 2.6 per cent of all hospital births. The percentage of births attended and the number of midwives practicing has been steadily increasing since the mid-1970s. The percentage of births at home or in birth centers has remained fairly constant at around 3 per cent of all births from 1980 to 1985. Midwives could do more and are looking at various ways to increase their usefulness.

Meetings have been held with state and county health officials to encourage the employment of midwives and improve reimbursement for midwives now providing care to low-income women. Midwives participate in public events with exhibits which promote their services. They also speak to school and community groups about childbirth and what midwives have to offer. Efforts are underway to increase ties with other groups interested in improving maternal-child health through coalitions which target specific problems such as teen pregnancy. In 1987 the Midwives Association organized a major statewide conference on birth-related public policy issues which was attended by a variety of practitioners, government officials, scholars and others concerned about the complex issues encountered in the organization of our maternity services.

We expect these activities to show results over time. It is important to recognize that there won't be an overnight change in the status of midwifery. However, if we remain united in our goal and have the strength to persist in our work, then it is quite possible that our daughters will come of age in a society where high-quality midwifery care is widely available.

NOTES

1 National Center for Health Statistics, Advance Report of Final Natality Statistics, *Monthly Vital Statistics Report*, vol. 36, no. 4, Supplement, July 1987.

2 Rooks, Judith and Haas, Eugene, *Nurse-Midwifery in America: A Report of the American College of Nurse-Midwives Foundation*, ACNM, 1986.

3 *Journal of Nurse-Midwifery*, vol. 29, no. 2, Special Legislative Issue, March/April 1984, pp. 55–174.

4 Myers, Susan, 'Midwifery in the United States: how regulations affect the profession,' unpublished paper, December 1986; 'Midwifery and the law,' *Mothering*, Special Edition, 1982.

5 Leavitt, Judith Walzer and Walton, Whitney, '"Down to death's door": women's perceptions of childbirth in America,' *Women and Health in America*, ed. Judith Walzer Leavitt, University of Wisconsin Press, 1984.

6 Leavitt, Judith Walzer, 'Birth and anesthesia: the debate over twilight sleep,' *Women and Health in America*, op. cit.

7 Wertz, Richard and Wertz, Dorothy, *Lying-In: A History of Childbirth in America*, Schocken Books, 1979.

8 Young, Diony (ed.), 'Obstetrical Intervention and Technology in the 1980s,' *Women and Health* 7(3/4), Haworth Press, 1983.

9 Guillemin, Jeanne Harley and Holmstrom, Lynda Lytle, 'The business of childbirth,' *American Hospital*, July/August 1986.

10 Litoff, Judy Barrett, *The American Midwife Debate: A Sourcebook on Its Modern Origins*, Greenwood Press, 1986; Litoff, Judy Barrett, *American Midwives: 1860 to the Present*, Greenwood Press, 1978; Devitt, Neal, 'The statistical case for the elimination of the midwife: fact versus prejudice, 1890–1935,' *Women and Health*, vol. 4, no. 1,

pp. 81–96 and vol. 4, no. 2, 1979, pp. 169–86; Speert, Harold, *Obstetrics and Gynecology in America*, American College of Obstetricians and Gynecologists, 1980.

11 Declercq, Eugene and Lacroix, Richard, 'The immigrant midwives of Lawrence: the conflict between law and culture in early twentieth-century Massachusetts,' *Bulletin of the History of Medicine*, vol. 59, pp. 232–46, 1985.

12 Taffel, Selma, *Midwife and Out-of-Hospital Deliveries, United States*, data from the National Vital Statistics System, series 21, no. 40, Public Health Service, Washington, DC, Government Printing Office, February 1984.

13 Hogan, Aileen, 'A tribute to the pioneers,' *Journal of Nurse-Midwifery*, reprint, Summer 1975.

14 Tom, Sally Austen, 'The evolution of nurse-midwifery: 1900–1960,' *Journal of Nurse-Midwifery*, vol. 27, no. 4, July/August 1982, pp. 4–13.

15 Thomas, Margaret W., *The Practice of Nurse-Midwifery in the United States*, US Department of Health, Education and Welfare, Children's Bureau, 1965.

16 Levy, Barry S., Wilkinson, Frederick, and Marine, William, 'Reducing neonatal mortality rates with nurse-midwives,' *American Journal of Obstetrics and Gynecology*, vol. 109, no. 1, January 1971, pp. 50–8.

17 *The Midwife in the United States: Report of a Macy Conference*, Josiah Macy, Jr Foundation, 1968.

18 Edwards, Margot and Waldorf, Mary, *Reclaiming Birth: History and Heroines of American Childbirth Reform*, Crossing Press, 1984.

19 Starr, Paul, *The Social Transformation of American Medicine*, Basic Books, 1982.

20 Boston Women's Health Book Collective, *Our Bodies, Our Selves*, Simon & Schuster, 1971.

21 Rothman, Barbara Katz, *In Labor: Women and Power in the Birthplace*, W.W. Norton, 1982.

22 Burst, Helen Varney, 'Two roads – which one?,' *Journal of Nurse-Midwifery*, vol. 26, no. 5, September/October 1981, pp. 7–12; Kreinberg, Nancy and McSweeney, Maryellen, 'An attitude survey of lay-midwives and nurse-midwives,' *Journal of Nurse-Midwifery*, vol. 26, no. 3, May/June 1981, pp. 43–50.

23 Charvet, Teddy, 'History of MANA,' *MANA News*, vol. 1, no. 1, Supplement, July 1983.

24 DeVries, Raymond, *Regulating Birth: Midwives, Medicine and the Law*, Temple University Press, 1985; see also Viewpoint Column in *MANA News*, 1984–87.

25 Adams, Constance, 'Management of delivery by United States

certified nurse-midwives,' *Journal of Nurse-Midwifery*, vol. 30, no. 1, January/February 1985, pp. 3–8.

26 Dempkowsky, Alfreda, 'Future prospects of nurse-midwifery in the United States,' *Journal of Nurse-Midwifery*, vol. 27, no. 2, March/April 1982, pp. 9–15; *Alternative Birthing Methods Study*, State of California, Office of Statewide Health Planning and Development, Legislative Report, Sacramento, California, 1986; Richmond, Julie and Wise, Paul, 'Midwifery and medicine in America: the struggle for justice in infant health,' *Journal of Nurse-Midwifery*, vol. 31, no. 5, September/October 1986, pp. 219–23.

27 Disbrow, Mildred (ed.), *Meeting Consumer's Demands for Maternity Care*, Proceedings of a Conference for Nurses and Other Health Professionals, University of Washington, Seattle, September 1972.

28 *Midwifery Outside of the Nursing Profession: The Current Debate in Washington*, Health Policy Analysis Program, School of Public Health and Community Medicine, University of Washington, Seattle, 1980.

29 Baird, Jane Elizabeth, 'A demographic study of Washington State licensed midwives,' unpublished thesis, School of Public Health and Community Medicine, University of Washington, Seattle, 1987.

INTRODUCTION
AUSTRALIA

When the first convict ships sailed into Sydney harbour in 1788 they brought with them women who served their sister convicts as midwives. The first maternity hospital was the Female Factory at Parramatta where women convicts were incarcerated. When transportation of female convicts stopped in 1848 this and other institutions like it were handed over to the local authorities.

Free settlers, in contrast, usually gave birth at home assisted by neighbours, or a granny, or a convict midwife. In South Australia they were often helped by Aboriginal women who used the skills handed down in their own culture.

Throughout the nineteenth century and into the twentieth a midwife came to the expectant mother's house shortly before the baby was due, lived with and got to know her, cared for her during labour, and stayed for some weeks after till she was fit and confident. By the close of the century midwifery training had been introduced in some parts of Australia and the first small maternity homes and specialised hospitals were opened.

As in other countries, the Second World War brought an enormous upheaval and a new style of obstetrics was introduced with strong American influence. By 1950 there was close on 100 per cent hospital birth, and all but a few midwives were also trained nurses. Fifteen years later there was no longer any provision for direct-entry midwifery.

The new Australian way of birth was hospital-centred, authoritarian, hierarchical and punitive in style – perhaps not so very different in atmosphere from that of the female convict factory. Babies were separated from their mothers and could only be viewed through glass by fathers and other members of the family. Children were not allowed to visit their mothers in hospital. Strict feeding schedules were insisted on and when women broke the rules they were treated like recalcitrant children. The first hospital to switch to rooming-in did so with the explanation that it was necessary because there had been an outbreak of staphylococcus in the newborn nursery.

The early 1970s saw the introduction of active management of labour by obstetricians, with routine intervention and liberal use of drugs. Obstetricians were the sole arbiters of care in childbirth and expected midwives to serve as their assistants or as temporary stand-ins during uneventful births.

Today many Australian midwives accept such a system more or less uncritically, but there is a growing movement for midwives to redefine their role in relation to the women they serve, as well as to general nurses and to obstetricians. Midwives are criticising the hospital system because it rarely allows them to give any continuity of care, and some point out that the introduction of new technology means that the midwife now has three 'patients' between which her attention must be uneasily divided – the mother, the foetus, and the machine.[1]

In this chapter a midwife analyses the present situation of Australian midwives and makes suggestions for urgent and much-needed changes.

NOTE

1   W. McDonald and J. Davis, *History of Midwifery Practice in Australia and the Western Pacific Regions.* Western Australian Branch of the National Midwives Association of Australia, for the 20th Congress of the International Confederation of Midwives, Sydney, 1984.

AUSTRALIAN MIDWIFERY TRAINING AND PRACTICE*

LESLEY BARCLAY

The National Midwives' Association of Australia adopted the World Health Organisation definition of a midwife (see page ix) in 1981. Paradoxically, the rules and regulations set out in most state ordinances do not appear to permit its implementation. Each state has its own idiosyncratic approach. Three states' regulations have neither definition, description of midwifery nor role limits. Most bear no resemblance to one another or to the World Health Organisation definition.

This chapter examines the regulations that control practice in Australia and the consequences of a lack of a strong, agreed national policy or standard for midwives.

BACKGROUND

Historically, midwives fulfilled the full breadth of the WHO definition. In New South Wales they cared for the majority of women well after the turn of the century and were still caring for 18 per cent in the late 1930s. They were demonstrably at least as safe as, and probably more so than, their medical colleagues.[1]

There is a paradox in that today's midwife, far better educated than her pre-war sister, is losing all vestiges of her independence.[2] Why did this happen? Despite the good performance of

* This is an edited version of a paper originally published in *Midwifery* (1985) no. 1. © Longman Group, 1985

early Australian midwives, Australians began to believe that doctors provided a superior service. We continued to pay them for their attendance, and our developing medical insurance systems did not recognise the midwife's role in delivery and furthered the medical profession's interests.[3]

Australia's situation is unique (apart from the United States) in the power exerted by private medical practice.[4] Doctors have status not accorded their overseas colleagues, and form the upper class in a peculiarly egalitarian society.[5] Nurses and midwives were recognised by medical practitioners as potential competitiors a hundred years ago.[6] To survive, they were forced to make concessions and to adopt a feminine subservience that sits uncomfortably with today's women.

Sexism combines powerfully with professional elitism and the fear of economic competition to assert medicine's dominance over less prestigious female health care workers.[7] Today's arguments for medical dominance in obstetrics rarely mention economic considerations. Earlier writers were either more perspicacious or less careful in masking their motives.

Despite their inability or intention to deliver all women, including those unable to pay, medical practitioners fought strongly against the training, registration, and even the existence of midwives in Australia. Forster makes this explicit:

> Doctor pre-eminence in obstetrics was continued by the medical profession's failure to provide any systematic training of midwives. There were heated arguments over what form training, if instituted, should take, because many doctors feared that the fully qualified midwife would not only take over obstetrical practice, but also invade the lucrative field of diseases of women.[8]

Such arguments were eventually overcome and a form of midwifery training began a little over a century ago. These training programmes accommodated both non-nurse and nurse entrants.

A tradition arose early this century in Australia that midwifery was necessary to complete one's training as a 'nurse'. It became an essential prerequisite for promotion.

Hospitals that offered midwife-only training tended to follow the English trend of setting lower entrance requirements. 'Direct-entry' training produced graduates who were less useful in our small cottage hospitals so important before the Second World War. These small district or country hospitals fulfilled both the medical and midwifery needs of the area. They required their limited staff to be able to meet any emergency. Therefore, a 'midwife' was limited in function where a 'nurse-midwife' was not. Conversely, a general nurse was also limited in such situations, as the major nurse training schools did not turn out nurses with even limited experience in midwifery. The era of the cottage hospitals disappeared as they were increasingly unable to meet the costs of advancing technology considered necessary for modern medicine.[9] Priorities in nursing training have altered in Australia though we still seem to hold a pre-war notion that the complete nurse must be a midwife also.

Because nurse training was, and generally at this time remains, different and separate from other forms of education available in the community, avenues for post-basic education have been very limited. This situation is rapidly changing with recent government policy stating that by the end of the 1980s all basic nurse training will be controlled by tertiary education systems, not individual hospitals. Promotion has been historically tied to one's ability to gain further certificates in nursing.

Changes in attitude and policies towards nurse education are having far-reaching consequences on the development of the profession. It is past time that the assumptions on midwifery education were questioned equally stringently and a similar re-examination of attitude and policy made.

Obviously, in our 'outback', nurse-midwives serve the community far more capably and at less cost than could be managed by a nurse and a midwife. The majority of nurses, however, are employed in areas where midwifery is required but irrelevant.[10] Limited opportunities for employment exist currently for any woman seeking to use midwifery and nursing together. Smaller country hospitals provide the most obvious examples of these. With extensive regionalisation of medical services, such hospitals are becoming less common.

THE FUNCTION OF THE MIDWIFE

'What is a midwife?' and 'What does a midwife do?' In different parts of Australia there would be different answers to these questions. No matter where she works, the midwife manages labour (but not necessarily delivery) and immediate post-natal care. A minority of midwives fill the WHO defined role – and more – in isolated areas. But it is very different for the majority of midwives, who work where medical services are amply provided.

Kilver's thorough study of midwives and doctors in two obstetric hospitals in Sydney found that the most highly qualified persons do not necessarily provide the best services.[11] Midwives regularly perform tasks below their level of training. Pupil midwives are consistently doing chores that could be equally well undertaken by less qualified persons and that have no educational component at all.

The outstanding and consistent feature of Kilver's and studies in other countries is the finding that midwifery skills are frequently underutilised and that as a result midwives are dissatisfied. Social, political and economic systems have impinged further and further on to midwifery in Australia, so there is very little remaining independent territory for the midwife, except in a subsidiary role. Notable exceptions are the relatively few midwives who work in the home birth movement and those in isolated outback regions.

Our health care systems are dominated by medical practitioners. Society has accorded them the right not only to this control, but also to define the needs of the market place.[12] This combination of social and economic control makes their political influence extremely powerful and difficult to counter.

THE REGULATION OF THE MIDWIFE

Australian midwives have lost their own regulatory bodies, which were formed after the turn of the century, to the nurses' registration boards (NRB) formed during the years 1920–1933.[13] These combined boards in no formal way protect the representation or rights of midwives.

It is possible to compare the legal function of the midwife in each state throughout pregnancy, labour and delivery and post-natally by examining the relevant regulations. We can also compare each definition with the WHO definition. Such a comparison demonstrates clearly that there are state differences of considerable magnitude. For example, midwives in Victoria are legally far more constrained in their role than those in New South Wales and Western Australia, and are confined to the auxiliary or assistant function. In the states midwives under-taking home birth do so with no guidelines or regulations governing their practice.

Perceptions of midwives and midwifery reflected in regula-tions are more likely to be those of nurses than of midwives themselves. The career structure that developed in nursing in the past has meant that many of our nursing leaders have, at the least, a limited view of midwifery. Midwives ambitious to further their careers frequently have to return to nursing to do so.

Australian midwifery had no spur to develop or maintain independence outside nursing. Willis, a sociologist, has produced convincing evidence to show that in Victoria nursing and medi-cine joined forces to reduce the independent practice of mid-wives.[14]

The formation of an active National Association of Midwives at the beginning of the 1980s suggests that midwives are capable of recognising their uniqueness and want to maintain a separate identity from nurses. It remains to be seen whether this move can lead to long overdue rethinking and revision of the mechanisms used to control midwifery practice.

DIRECT-ENTRY MIDWIFERY

Australian perception of non-nurse midwives is determined by professional memory and regionalised limited viewpoints.

'Direct-entry' courses (that is, training programmes in mid-wifery for non-nurses) were only discontinued in the 1970s. The Federal Government's Directory of Courses, 1966, shows all states offering two-year midwifery programmes. Subsequent publications no longer show basic courses, so one has to extrapo-late from these figures and those of *Nursing Personnel*, vol. II,

1979, which shows none trained in Australia after 1977. Some time over this decade the courses offered ceased.

Unfortunately, statistics showing the career pattern of these midwives are not available. It seems a reasonable assumption that motivation to work as a midwife is high in such candidates and that wastage rates of those who complete training is low. Overseas experience supports this.[15] Recent Australian work shows that where motivation of nurse candidates for midwifery training was not high wastage rates of recently trained midwives were nearly 50 per cent.[16] Increased cost-effectiveness of a longer training period for non-nurses appears not to be justifiable. The current system is not cost-effective and is wasteful of resources.[17] Australia is large enough to tolerate a two-tier system of training, and the benefits of a less mobile, highly motivated midwifery workforce could be considerable. The midwife who is not a registered nurse would face limitations of promotion within general hospital structures, but should not be limited within the area of midwifery itself. A longer training period would be necessary to ensure that standards were maintained. The National Midwives' Association supports such direct-entry training programmes. This development is consistent with recent moves in the United States.

The question of direct entry is not simple. It is an issue most Australian nurses have not considered except negatively. Yet it is one worthy of rethinking in the light of international development and the dubious cost-effectiveness of current training methods.

THE WASTAGE OF MIDWIFERY-TRAINED NURSES FROM MIDWIFERY PRACTICE

Nursing Personnel: A National Survey, published by the Commonwealth Department of Health (vol. I, 1979) showed alarming wastage of training facilities and resources in midwifery education. These findings are confirmed by more recent state enquiries held in New South Wales and South Australia.[18]

Over 2,000 midwives are trained annually, and yet of those sampled in a comprehensive national survey only 5,926 registered nurses (both registered midwives and midwifery students)

Table 1: Total registrants with midwifery certificates employed in areas where midwifery could contribute to performance

Areas		Numbers
Infant welfare		1,163
General community nurse		570
Paediatrics		574
Administration (excluding ward units)		1,772
Hospital-based nurse education		736
Midwifery-qualified nures working in related areas		3,815
Midwives employed in midwifery units		4,600
	Total	8,415
Total registrants holding midwifery certificates		37,746

Source: derived from figures taken from *Nursing Personnel: A National Survey*, Canberra, Commonwealth Department of Health, 1979.

were directly employed in midwifery.[19] An approximation derived from these figures puts the midwifery workforce in 1979 at about 6,800. When one subtracts the student workforce of approximately 2,200, the total number of trained midwives employed directly in midwifery is approximately 4,600.

It is acknowledged that of the 37,746 registrants holding a midwifery certificate,[20] many may find midwifery a desirable or necessary addition to their nursing qualification. If one totals, however, allied fields where midwifery could contribute to the quality of care delivered (even indirectly) and adds those nurses directly practising midwifery, only approximately one-quarter of those trained are in any way benefiting from their training (see Table 1). Conversely, their training is in no demonstrable way contributing to the quality of care within our health systems.

A review of British nursing and midwifery journals between 1980 and 1985 shows many articles directly related to dissatisfaction with current training programmes, concern for wise future development, current wastage of training opportunities, and the need to rethink a professional identity. A similar review of Australian journals shows very few that could be similarly classified. The lack of concern in Australia seems to reflect our perception of midwifery as an extension of nursing.

Fifty-five training schools across Australia produce approximately one-third of the total employed workforce annually. The expenditure on this training needs to be examined and justified, as:

(a) only 27 per cent of those undertaking training did so to be able to work as midwives; and

(b) only 56 per cent of those trained in 1981–82 were working in midwifery in 1984.[21]

It seems that Moore's suspicions that recruitment into midwifery training in the United Kingdom is not based on rational manpower planning holds in Australia also. He deplores the training of 4,000 midwives annually to replenish a pool of 20,000 employed. He sees this as a disproportionate investment in training.[22] Australia trains nearly one-third of its employed workforce annually, an even higher ratio.

NATIONAL POLICY

The lack of national policy for midwifery both contributes to and compounds problems faced in individual states. Australia as a nation has not identified the goals of midwifery. The midwife's function is not clearly defined in most states or comparable, legally at least, across all states. The National Midwives' Association, formed in 1977, is grappling with many of these issues and developing its own policy. The growth and strength of this group was evident to midwives from around the world when they attended the International Congress in Sydney in 1984. The implementation of policy requires an equal concern and commitment from government and statutory bodies that control the profession.

CONCLUSION

Midwifery's practice and development have been retarded by its retention of nineteenth-century models of subservience to males and medical practice and its acceptance of a 'delicacy of female intellect'.[23] This has been compounded by the incorporation of midwifery into nursing. 'Midwifery changed its structural location within the health division of labour from an independent status to a subordinate one.'[24]

The unsophisticated acceptance of a patently questionable system of midwifery education can be demonstrated quantitatively.[25] Some states' attempts to regulate practice are antiquated and of dubious worth. Most show a deference to medical nursing controls that were established and are maintained on grounds that are clearly open to challenge.

The lack of concern expressed on these issues in Australia reflects our perceptions of midwifery as an extension of nursing and our acceptance that nursing leadership is fitting, appropriate and satisfactory for midwifery. I seriously question those assumptions and demonstrate that this has not proved adequate in the past. The majority of midwives today are performing tasks not seen as advantageous, desirable or economically rewarding by other groups. As a consequence, the midwife as a strong practitioner with respected opinions and a high degree of skill is in danger of disappearing. Domination of midwifery by medicine has been abetted, albeit unintentionally, by the close links between nursing and midwifery in this country.[26]

Discussions at an international level, for example at Council Meetings of the International Confederation of Midwives, indicate that erosion of practice is not just an Australian issue. Other nations, despite their more auspicious beginnings, are experiencing a similar phenomenon. The breadth of this challenge requires international response, support and action.

Only through midwives' own commitment and enthusiasm nationally and internationally can we meet this challenge. I have no doubt that the abundance of talent, skills and determination of midwives will win out in the end.

NOTES

1   M.J. Lewis, 'Obstetric education and practice in Sydney 1870–1930: Part I', *The Australian and New Zealand Journal of Obstetrics and Gynaecology*, vol. 18, no. 3, August 1978; N. Williamson, 'She walked . . . with Great Purpose', in M. Bevenge *et al.* (eds), *Worth Her Salt: Women at Work in Australia*, Hale & Iremonger, 1982.

2   W. Adcock *et al.*, *With Courage and Devotion: A History of Midwifery*

in *New South Wales*, New South Wales Midwives' Association, 1984.

3 T.S. Pensabene, *The Rise of the Medical Practitioner in Victoria*, Australian National University Press, 1980.

4 R.B. Scotton, *Medical Care in Australia: An Economic Diagnosis*, Sun Books for the Institute of Applied Economic and Social Research, University of Melbourne, 1974.

5 Pensabene, op. cit.

6 F.M.C. Forster, *Progress in Obstetrics and Gynaecology in Australia*, John Sands, 1967.

7 E. Willis, *Medical Dominance*, Allen & Unwin, 1983.

8 Forster, op. cit., p. 15.

9 A. Thornton, 'The past in midwifery services', *Australia Nurses Journal*, March 1972, pp. 19–23.

10 See *Nursing Personnel: A National Survey*, Report of the Committee on Nursing, vols 1 and 2, Commonwealth Department of Health AGPS Canberra, 1979.

11 T. Kilver, *Task Analysis of Obstetric Care: An Investigation of the Health Services Mobility Study (Gilpatrick) Method*, Hospitals and Health Services Commission, New South Wales, 1976.

12 Scotton, op. cit.

13 T.J. Matson, 'Teaching Tomorrow's Midwives', *Australian Nurses Journal*, vol. 7, no. 6, 1978, pp. 41–4.

14 Willis, op. cit.

15 H.G. Ball, 'Direct-entry midwives: a special class', *Midwives Chronicle and Nursing Notes*, 1982, pp. 12–13.

16 L.M. Barclay, 'An enquiry into midwives' perceptions of the training', *Australian Journal of Advanced Nursing*, vol. 1, no. 4, 1984, pp. 11–23.

17 Ibid.

18 V. Bayliss, *Midwifery Manpower Study*, Health Commission of New South Wales, 1981; J. Beecken, *Specific Issues Relating to Midwifery*, Stage 2 of the Nursing Manpower Study, South Australian Health Commission and Nurses' Board of South Australia, Adelaide, 1981.

19 *Nursing Personnel*, op. cit.

20 Ibid.

21 Barclay, op. cit.

22 B. Moores, 'Towards rational midwifery service planning', *Journal of Advanced Midwifery*, vol. 5, 1980, pp. 301–11.

23 G. Law, '"I have never liked trade unionism": the development of the Royal Australian Nursing Federation, Queensland Branch, 1904–45', in E. Windshuttle (ed.), *Women, Class and History*, Fontana/Collins, 1980.

24 Willis, op. cit., p. 93.
25 Barclay, op. cit.
26 Willis, op. cit.

INTRODUCTION

CANADA

Since the late nineteenth century midwifery has been illegal in most provinces of Canada. In not having an organised midwifery system Canada has ranked internationally along with Panama, El Salvador, Venezuela, Colombia, Honduras, the Dominican Republic and Burundi.

Care in childbirth is compartmentalised. Pregnancy is overseen by an obstetrician. A case room obstetric nurse takes orders from the obstetrician and cares for the woman when she is in labour. A nursery nurse takes orders from the paediatrician in caring for the newborn baby. A postpartum nurse cares for the woman after delivery, also under the direction of the obstetrician. And once the mother and baby are home, care is divided between a paediatrician, a general practitioner physician, and a public health nurse.

Pressure for change has come from the home birth movement. This process started in the mid-1970s with the rebirth of a legally recognised community midwifery in isolated places in British Columbia, Alberta, Saskatchewan, Ontario and the Maritimes. In the 1980s there was a great deal of publicity surrounding inquests on two babies who had died following midwife care. This resulted, not in the condemnation of midwives as might be expected, but in a recommendation that a programme for the study of midwifery, leading to a licence to practise midwifery, should be set up by the College of Physicians and Surgeons. It was also recommended that midwifery be legalised in Ontario, and that the profession be recognised and incorporated as an integral part of the Ontario health care system, covered by health care insurance. This was followed in January 1986 by an announcement by the Minister of Health that, 'It is our government's intention to establish midwifery as a recognised part of the Ontario Health Care System,' and the subsequent setting up of a Midwifery Task Force to explore ways in which midwives should be trained and registered, and how they should work.

In this chapter Jutta Mason looks at the history of midwifery in Canada and sees first how midwifery was destroyed, and then how it has been recreated.

MIDWIFERY IN CANADA

*JUTTA MASON**

When women and men from France, the British Isles, and elsewhere in Europe left their homelands during the last two centuries and migrated in large numbers to Canada, the requirements of this new land resulted in major changes in their way of living. The manner of giving birth was one thing that changed for them immediately. Although many of the earlier settlers in Canada came from countries where doctors had already come to be regarded as appropriate birth attendants to the middle class, when these settlers arrived in the North American wilderness, they adapted themselves very quickly to the needs of their new situation and recast their birth culture to one of family and neighbour involvement. The sharing of the birth event must have been an important factor in strengthening family bonds in this foreign land, and in establishing emotional links between the groups of randomly assembled, often homesick, strangers as they began to form their new communities.

The midwives who developed from this neighbourly birth culture rarely made birth their profession. Although midwives in Ville-Marie (now Montreal) were elected by the women of the community and salaried by the French king from the beginning of the eighteenth century until the English conquest in 1759, and the British government briefly paid wages for midwives in Nova Scotia from 1755 to 1764, official recognition and support of midwives were otherwise lacking in Canada's history. Nor could most midwives make a living selling their services privately. The

* A longer version of the first two-thirds of this chapter has appeared as an 'Appendix on the history of midwifery in Canada' in the 1987 Ontario government publication, *Report of the Task Force on the Implementation of Midwifery in Ontario*. I would like to thank three women for their help: Catherine Penz, Jane Corcoran and Holiday Tyson.

population was widely scattered and currency was scarce. Doctors had the same problem in most parts of Canada until the end of the nineteenth century.

The settlers who arrived from Europe thus found that they had to look after themselves in childbirth. Mary O'Brien lived north of York (Toronto) and kept a journal from 1828 to 1838. She reported to her family back in England that, since the doctor lived so far away and didn't get there on time, her husband was her most important assistant at the birth of her daughter:

> It was with more cheerfulness than awe that, with occasional interruptions and the assistance of the damsel [servant] I arranged my bed. . . . I was secretly rejoicing in the probability of being beforehand with the doctor. I then methodically, with Edward's assistance, undressed and prepared myself. I placed everything likely to be wanted within reach. . . . In about ten minutes after, and almost as soon as I became assured that the crisis of my complaint was actually coming on, the little damsel was in her father's hands, audibly existent. In two minutes more she was lying snugly in my arms till the conclusion of our operations should give us leisure to attend to her further needs.[1]

The placenta was slow in coming, but was delivered after an hour, during which the baby spent her time nursing at her mother's breast. When everything was done, the doctor arrived 'to congratulate us, eat his supper, and go to bed'. This was Mary O'Brien's third child. She had had a doctor at the births of the first two, but seems to have felt no need of one from then on. A month afterwards, she got word that she should go and help another woman:

> Nov. 15 – a fine day. I was arranging to pay a visit to the shanties when I was sent for to the assistance of one of our labourers' wives on the wharf. I packed up my baby in the arms of my damsel whom I needed as interpreter and, leaving the other two with Edward, I hastened away. I arrived just in time to do the needful for a fine little girl. This is the second time I have cheated the doctor in four weeks. The said doctor arrived just after the work was done to look very foolish and

go home with me to dine (said doctor not being the same whom I cheated before). He is a young Scotsman lately come out. Doctors have no chance at such work here. We make so light of it.[2]

Mary O'Brien's account makes it clear that some settlers came to see their enforced self-reliance in childbirth as a positive benefit.

Helping out at births was something that neighbours did for one another. There was often a woman with extra skill and experience, who might be especially sought out when a woman was in labour, but these special women rarely did more than sixty to ninety births during their lifetime. Sometimes they owned fat household-veterinary-medical books where they could look up instructions if they needed to. Some had brought seeds from their home country and planted a medicinal herb garden. Their primary function was running their own households, however, and in rural areas that meant they were very occupied indeed. Their training thus consisted not of years of study and apprenticeship, but of their participation in a culture in which most adult women expected to have to help one another at the time of birth.

At the margins of settlements the distance between the homes was sometimes so great that a woman might have only her husband or even her oldest daughter as her birth assistant. If the husband was off trapping or hunting, it was not uncommon for the woman to be quite alone when she went into labour. But such a situation was not seen as desirable. Whenever possible, women were joined by female neighbours and relatives when they gave birth. There is little mention of special techniques used by these women as they helped one another. They seem to have interfered very little. The one main, overriding rule seems to have been to stay with the mother throughout the whole of her labour, to comfort her and never to leave her by herself:

I mean, we didn't know exactly when a baby was going to be born, but when you were there, you just didn't feel like leaving. The mother was more reassured when you were with them, you know. And you weren't always doing a lot of work all the hours previous to the birth of the child, but you were doing anything you could to allay fears, perhaps for a young mother with her first child. They had to be comforted. And you know, just the little things – if you only rub their back a bit or things like that, they'd help a bit, you see?[3]

Position in labour varied. Most women tried to walk around and keep to their activities as long as possible during the first part of their labour, and squatting seems to have been common during the pushing stage. There is seldom mention of the boiling of instruments or the preparing of sterile cloths until the 1940s. The theories of Semmelweiss and Lister about invisible contamination found little application in the popular birth culture. Nevertheless, infection seems to have been rare. It was seen as important to keep clean. Some women made themselves a little mattress of 'the cleanest straw' and delivered their baby on to that.

It was the custom in all but the most isolated areas to insist on three to ten days' rest for the new mother, during which time she might get up to go to the outhouse or to take meals with the family, but had otherwise to stay in bed 'to let everything settle back into place'. At a time when the workload of the farm woman extended from before dawn to late evening, such a break must have been spiritually as well as physically profoundly helpful. The material aid given to the household at the time after birth by the neighbour women was seen as being of equal importance to the supportive circle during the birth. The women who waited on the mother afterwards travelled back and forth between the home of the new mother and their own homes, where their work still had to be done. If a project was underway when the call came that a woman was in labour, that project might be brought along:

I recall one time a man coming 18 miles in a sleigh to take my grandmother to his wife who was expecting a baby. My grandmother had mixed bread dough earlier in the day, so she packed the pan of dough in with her in this sleigh, which was comfortably warm with lots of blankets and quilts and heated stones. When she arrived at the farmer's home the dough had risen enough to bake, so she baked it in the stove in his kitchen, and after she delivered the baby, the husband drove my grandmother home with her bread baked.[4]

So the baby was born and the bread was done. Having a baby, while it was seen as a very special occasion, did not involve a radical break from the business of daily life. Even the trained nurses who later on came to work in outpost communities seem to have soon abandoned much of the bustling and sterilizing and graphing that they had been taught at their nursing schools. The event of birth was so securely entwined with the other work of women – the preparation of food, the manufacturing of clothing, the maintaining of the home – that the nurses might find themselves pulled into the female activities surrounding the birth. Here is an account by nurse Myra Bennett of a birth she attended in Labrador:

> I remember on one occasion I was attending a maternity case some miles away from home. It was a first baby and didn't seem to be in a particular hurry to arrive. Everything was normal but we didn't feel right about going to bed, when the patient was experiencing discomfort, so we got to work. . . . The father-in-law was a fisherman who needed new mitts, so out came the bag of wool. . . . [After the carding and spinning were done] one of the younger girls commenced to knit the mitts, and during that night of waiting, a brand new pair of mittens were completed for the thankful father.
>
> In between the spinning and completion of the mitts I had set to work cooking up a huge pot of stew. We prepared fresh rabbits, some salt beef, all the vegetables obtainable . . . and these were cooked together until they were almost tender enough to fall apart. It was an absolutely delicious stew. . . . The patient commenced the more urgent stage of her labour well fortified with this meal, and we who attended her had a very satisfactory night which ended in the morning with the arrival of a perfectly beautiful baby.[5]

A primary characteristic of the popular birth culture was that the birthing woman was surrounded by other women whom she knew, who shared her life and fate and status in most respects and who expected to fit themselves to the needs of the new baby's family rather than imposing any medical structure on the event. It appears that money was seldom exchanged for this kind of help. 'Turnabout' help was the labour that tied the new communities together and enabled them to be built up from nothing in a relatively short time. Help at birth times would generally be repaid with produce or with help with farm work, housework, or birth attendance at a different house the next season.

Although non-interference seems to have been the practice at most births, the birth culture did have resources to deal with difficulties if they came up. They may not have come up all that often – settlers' accounts often stress their good health: 'Women in them days, they worked hard and it didn't bother them any.' Birth lore held that a woman who was pregnant ought to eat plenty of good food without restriction, and to carry on being physically active until her labour began.

If problems did arise, the story told by nurse Myra Bennett (about the rabbit stew which fortified a woman whose labour was slow) illustrates a gentle folk remedy for a mother who might be running out of energy during her labour. The efficacy of the preparation of food, its value not only as sustenance but also as a loving gift from one person to another, seems to have been understood and used often in the popular birth culture. When doctors and nurses first came to work with the people of the isolated areas, they sometimes adapted this humble technique. Nurse Jo Lutley tells how she learned about the therapeutic value of food from another physician:

When I went to the Grenfell Mission on the Labrador coast, I was told how Dr Grenfell, when he went up the coast and was called in to do a delivery, and it took a long time, and the mother seemed to be getting tired and she didn't seem to be getting anywhere, he would say, 'Ah, well, I think I'll cook you up something to eat.' And he'd perhaps get out some eggs and bacon. In those days, in many of the homes he went into, that would have been a great luxury. And so he would start cooking that up for the mother. And the story goes that more often than not, before he had finished cooking it in readiness for her, maybe the good smells of it or something, she would go into active labour and deliver. And so I've always gone on that same kind of thing.[6]

Some remedies, although gentle, were active measures to forestall a potential crisis. If a crisis became more acute, more vigorous measures were employed. An example is the practice of 'quilling', in which the midwife would put some cayenne pepper into a hollowed-out goose quill and blow it into the nose of a woman who seemed to be making no progress pushing her baby out. A doctor who watched a midwife do this wrote an account of the experience.

> [The labouring woman] began to sneeze immediately. With the sneezing the midwife said, 'Doc, you'd better get ready.'
> By the time I had taken a look at things, the perineum was bulging, and with another few sneezes, the baby was born. The midwife made only this remark, 'I knew, Doc, that this would make her let go her 'holt.' I have never forgotten this way of conducting a quick labour.[7]

In the case of a dire emergency such as a woman in convulsions with eclampsia, treatments mentioned in early accounts included hot water compresses, bleeding, and rubbing the woman all over with wet towels. The factor common to all accounts was the constant, assiduous attention paid to the mother. Sometimes both mother and baby survived. If a baby was wedged in because of a transverse lie or disproportion, the midwife resorted to dismemberment, as did the doctors of that time – with the difference that the doctors had special instruments and chloroform to mask the process from the mother, while the midwife had to pull the baby out piece by piece from the uterus of a conscious mother. Such occasions, although widely publicised in medical stories about midwives, seem to have been uncommon.

The few maternal mortality studies investigating medically unserviced areas in Canada (none was done before 1918) startled the investigators by their superior outcomes. Dr M. Seymour, Medical Officer of Health for Saskatchewan, reported at a meeting of the Saskatchewan Medical Association in 1919 that the 50 per cent of the province's women who gave birth without either doctor or nurse attending had a 'much lower' maternal mortality than the other 50 per cent. The reaction to his announcement was not positive:

> I was very strongly taken to task by some of the members for even compiling these figures. I told them I thought the proper

place to give these figures was to a meeting of medical men. I was taking care that they were not being published.[8]

Similar results were reported in Manitoba during the 1920s.[9] In Ontario, an investigation in 1928 by the Ontario Red Cross, in which they sought statistical evidence of the advantage of having Red Cross hospitals in isolated areas, came up with the disappointing information that maternal mortality in Red Cross hospitals was higher than in medically unserviced areas. In fact, when maternal mortality figures of five large unserviced areas were averaged, they were lower than maternal mortality for Ontario as a whole (4.3 per 1,000 as against 5.6 per 1,000).[10]

None of the surveys indicating superior outcomes for undoctored births was followed up. By the turn of the century, when the popular birth culture was still highly developed, there was already a growing belief in the superiority of medical birth, especially on the part of investigators with a medical education. The proponents of more extensive medical involvement in birth had no interest in documenting the positive attributes of the traditional birth culture.

Towards the end of the nineteenth century, as the population increased considerably through immigration, and the number of doctors multiplied, midwives came into disfavour with physicians. Since the doctors were well connected with the government in all parts of the country, they had no difficulty in appropriating birth to their profession and making the popular birth culture illegal. But because neighbourly birth help was so widespread, it was almost impossible to single out midwives for prosecution. Attempts to take individual women to court met with strong popular resistance and uncooperative judges.[11] Even so, the pressure by the medical profession began to take its toll. Dr Benjamin Atlee of Halifax, reminiscing about his long career in obstetrics in eastern Canada, recalled how the last midwife he knew had been pressurised by local doctors to stop working:

She had a place where she took the better class of unmarried women . . . and she delivered them. But the profession ganged up on her – every step she made was watched like a hawk. . . . They thought they were losing money. The midwives would take money away from them. And then, of course, there was the all-abiding anti-feminism. How can a woman deliver a baby, sort of thing. . . . They tried to hit her for malpractice but they couldn't do it. She gave up – she was the last one. [12]

Direct pressure on neighbour birth helpers was augmented by increasing numbers of articles in magazines and public statements by doctors on the dangers of non-medical birth. Paradoxically, medical efforts to spread the message that childbirth needed to be handled by someone with special training contributed to the creation, in 1897, of a new movement that threatened the doctors' prospects for hegemony over birth more directly than any aspect of the existing birth culture. The movement was the formation of the Victorian Order of Home Helpers, by the National Council of Women of Canada. 'Women who have already lived in the country districts and who are respected, and have the confidence of their neighbours' were to be trained for six months to a year, primarily in midwifery but also in first aid, simple nursing, and 'household economy and sanitation'. [13]

The society ladies who belonged to the National Council of Women sought to connect the neighbourly birth culture with the benefits of medical obstetrics, already advertised to be safer and more progressive by the medical professon. Nurses, the new medical auxiliaries then beginning to carve out a role for themselves, were seen by the National Council as unsuitable maternity assistants because they were too bound by their rules and their routines. 'The need was . . . for a practical woman who has some training and will go from house to house doing all sorts of mercy and kindnesses, rather than the nurse just selected to go to a certain place to attend a certain case.' Doing favours 'turnabout', as we have seen, was an important part of farming life in Canada. The National Council of Women now wished to institutionalise this part of women's culture. The Home Helpers were to be women who were not only trained in the medical method of childbirth but who were also prepared to help muck out the barn and do the washing up while the new mother was still resting after the birth. No one claimed that the Home Helpers would be equivalent to the physician in their ability to handle births, but it was felt that they would be an ideal interim worker to service rural areas whose populations were still too scattered and too poor in currency to be able to support a doctor.

The members of the National Council of Women, having devised a plan to give existing neighbour birth helpers some of the additional training that doctors said was necessary, were startled and dismayed to find that, as soon as their plan became public, medical opposition was virtually unanimous. The trained nurses were the first to object publicly. Their efforts to gain economic security had centred around their campaign to gain public recognition for trained nurses as the only legitimate auxiliaries to doctors. A new type of worker with a shorter training and probably lower wages than those required by urban nurses would undermine the nurses' project to gain a secure profession. Pressure from the trained nurses was so strong that the National Council of Women made a radical change in their conception of the new organisation. Instead of using local women who were already established birth helpers they agreed to hire only trained nurses.

Far from reducing medical opposition to the organisation, this move even intensified it. Doctors charged that the Victorian Order of Nurses would 'ruin the young doctors and the country doctors, as the people would send for the nurses instead of them'. Reassurances that the Victorian Order would work mainly in areas where there was no doctor made no impression. The problem was clearly that midwifery was about to become legitimised by being turned into a job. The spectre of the British midwife was raised at medical meetings. In Britain, 'good men were forced to make visits at a shilling each' to counter the competition of the midwives. The nurses of the Victorian Order, who were to earn their livelihood through midwifery, would need to be in direct competition with physicians in a way that neighbour helpers never were.

Medical opposition grew so strong that Lady Aberdeen, the head of the National Council of Women, and the wife of Canada's Governor-General, was advised by her committee to stop campaigning for the Victorian Order: 'the articles on the Order and on those promoting it had become so virulent that they felt the Governor General and his wife should not be exposed to such opposition.'[14] But Lady Aberdeen persisted. She finally sought help from an American physician, Dr Alfred Worcester, who ran the only non-hospital training school for district nurses in North America. Worcester advised the National

Council of Women to remove all talk of midwifery and to present the scheme as one of district nursing, with the nurse in strict obedience to the doctor and subject to instant dismissal if she took any action on her own. The National Council, rather than let their project die, acquiesced. Dr Worcester then lectured to medical societies all over eastern Canada. He assured them that the Victorian Order nurses would simply be efficient assistants in the home, making the doctor's work lighter and seeing to it that his orders were carried out.

Dr Worcester's lectures gradually obtained grudging support for the Victorian Order of Nurses from the majority of Canadian physicians. In January 1898, the Order was permitted to begin work, a shadow of its former conception, doing nursing in the urban poor areas for the most part.

Although Lady Aberdeen's grand plan to institutionalise the neighbour helper had only limited results, the popular birth culture seems to have been minimally affected by the plan's failure. Communities carried on much as they had prior to the National Council of Women initiative, gradually accommodating the rising number of doctors who declared their intention of taking a role in birth. Not infrequently, the country doctors started their careers by working with traditional birth helpers. Although nominally these local 'grannies' or 'handywomen' were the doctor's assistants, the very poor obstetrical training (observing four deliveries fulfilled the practical requirements) available in most medical schools until after the First World War meant that the new doctors had to observe local birth customs closely and to learn their trade in this setting. For some doctors their community apprenticeships influenced their practice for the rest of their lives. The first national maternal mortality survey in 1927 drew attention to the work of a number of country doctors who had unusually low mortality rates – and who on interview said they almost never used forceps nor many of the other drugs or disinfecting agents which had come into vogue in mainstream obstetrics by that time.[15] These doctors, although they may have been regarded as dinosaurs by their city colleagues, often came to be held in high regard in their own communities.

But not all doctors integrated themselves into local customs. When a new physician arrived in a community and expected to be able unilaterally to set the terms of his relationship with the people of the area, he could find himself rejected. Particularly contentious were the billing practices of doctors, who were not willing to provide housework or farm labour at the time of a birth, and who expected to be paid whether or not they had arrived at a birth in time to help, as the following account shows:

> After a while our family began to come along. . . . I'd never had a doctor ever since I'd come from England to Canada and then it wasn't because I wanted to but because they told me I should. . . . They told us you'll have to have a doctor. . . . So we sent for one and they was three hours late and I had everything done, had the baby dressed and myself washed and the afterbirth taken out and put into the heater. And then he came and felt my pulse and said, 'Well you're just as nature led you. That's forty-five dollars please.' Yes, that was it and he'd only come six miles. . . . But I had sent for him and naturally I had to pay him. So after that when I was in a family way I never sought for any doctor. I asked the Lord to help me and he gave me health and strength. I had all twelve of them without any doctor or woman. . . . But I will say, at this time, I saw an advertisement in the Free Press about Indians using herbs to cut down labor pains and they were a dollar a box. So I thought, well I'll send for a box anyway. And as soon as the labor pains started I took a cupful of these herbs that was steeped in water and that took out all the labor pains. . . . And the last baby that was born, I stood up and caught him in my arms and laid him on the bed and reached over and got the scissors and separated the cord. Then I got a bowl of warm water and washed him and fixed up myself.[16]

Some women returned to their own resources after trying out doctors at their births. Women's scepticism about the claims of medical obstetrics resulted in financial hardship for physicians and underutilisation of clinics and cottage hospitals in areas where the popular birth culture was well-developed.

In the years immediately after the First World War, the much enlarged profession of trained nursing therefore threw its impressive energies into the campaign to convert women to medical birth. The nurses' proselytising role was one consequence of their continuing difficulties in finding work.

Hospitals still did not hire back their graduates, preferring the economies of using free student labour. The new career of public health nursing, which provided nurses with a government salary for working with sick people or pregnant women in their homes, offered a solution for underemployment of nurses.

But this solution had its own difficulties. Public health nurses encountered great hostility from doctors, who felt that nurses working outside of hospital supervision might encroach on medical prerogatives. The direct nursing and childbirth care that the nurses originally hoped to undertake thus gave way in many areas to a very strictly defined 'health teaching' role. Nurses sought to win over the doctors to the usefulness of their function by becoming outspoken advocates of doctor-managed birth and health care. In this capacity they worked tirelessly, visiting homes, schools, church and women's group meetings, handing out pamphlets and advice. Besides mentioning the illegality of the midwife, the text of these pamphlets took a tone new to the childbirth culture, emphasising that the labouring woman could now yield up her own responsibility and depend on her birth assistants to take care of her totally:

> The doctor will relieve you of pain as much as possible and will stay with you till you are quite safe. If this is not your first baby, it may not take more than one or two hours. Everybody will take care of you. The doctor and nurse will take charge of everything for you, till you and the baby are quite safe. And then you will have a good rest until you get your strength back.[17]

The federal government publication *The Canadian Mother's Book*, from which this excerpt was taken, had a run of more than a million copies before it was replaced by the next edition in 1940. Radio talks on the same subject reiterated the theme of birth as a time for the doctor to take over completely. Dr Roy Dafoe, a country doctor made famous because of his role as physician to the Dionne quintuplets,* had this to say in a very successful series of radio 'chats' of advice to women:

* The Dionne quintuplets were five identical girls born in 1934 in a remote farming area of northern Ontario. Dr Roy Dafoe arrived in time to deliver the last two quintuplets (the first three having been delivered by midwives) and for this he was proposed for the 1934 Nobel Prize in Medicine. The quintuplets quickly

During pregnancy: It is not necessary for me to remind you again that this is a time when you must place yourself unreservedly in the hands of your medical advisor, and when the best help you can give will be in the spirit of complete submission and co-operation. Remember that the various measures you will be asked to take are essential for your welfare and for the safety of your baby. The doctor knows by experience (and his own skill is backed up by all the accumulated wisdom of his profession) just what to do for you.[18]

The effect of this constant message was a gradual undermining of women's confidence in their own birth culture. Middle-class women began to regard the hospital as the appropriate place of birth, and of course the informal birth culture had no place at the hospital. There was a tendency for medical workers to congregate in urban centres, and although the message of the public health nurses, the advice books, magazine articles and radio broadcasts reached to the edges of settlement, the corresponding medical services did not. The effect was often the disintegration of the local birth culture, with no corresponding supply of doctors who would be willing to manage the births of those unable to afford their fees. Mrs Leonard Renaud, who lived in northern Ontario, wrote a letter to the Department of Health in Ottawa in 1935, reporting that doctors in her area had refused to attend at her births because she had not the twenty-five dollars to pay them. She, her husband, and a neighbour had managed the birth of twin boys without medical help. But they had derived no satisfaction from their success, having been convinced that such a birth was unnatural and 'a perfect disgrace'. Now she was pregnant again, and was appealing to the Department of Health for help:

Please tell me what I can do when my time is come this winter. Is there no doctors for the poor who will be paid by the Government for saving the mothers. . . . I have a little girl of four years past, born before we came here, then the two boys,

became world famous, and a 'hospital' was built for them by the government. There Dafoe supervised the scientific rearing of the quintuplets for the first six years of their lives, allowing their parents occasional visits. Hence his claim to expertise in childbirth and childrearing.

and my baby of last summer. There is no-one on this earth can care for these little ones like their own mother, and it would be terrible to have them handed into the care of others through neglect of me, the mother, at a most serious time. If I were strong I would try and face the next one as brave as we Canadian mothers are, but I fear I have not the strength nor the proper nourishment before time to enable me to stand it, without some aid.[19]

Mrs Renaud was in poor health because she was starving. There was no agency available to get her more food, and to ask for food would be begging, but to ask for medical aid was simply asking for the proper due of any mother. She had converted her need for food into the need for a doctor. But no doctor came. As local birth networks began to fade away, more and more women began to demand medical help, saying it was the responsibility of the government to do something to send medical workers into all parts of the country. In rural areas with scattered populations doctors could not make sufficient income, and so there came to be more nurses, on government salary, who came in preaching the gospel of medical birth and stayed to deliver the babies.

These nurses were never officially called midwives. They were sent by the Red Cross, the Victorian Order of Nurses, and provincial public health departments. Many of them were not well prepared but they learned on the job. Some were actually British trained midwives, but they did not advertise this fact. Attempts during the decade after the First World War by the head of the Victorian Order of Nurses, successive wives of Governors-General, and the Women's Grain Growers Association to introduce the trained midwife into Canada all failed. Although many nurses in outlying regions and even in urban poor areas did 'emergency' midwifery for women too remote, too poor or too unwilling to use doctors, this work was always referred to as 'maternity nursing' to avoid a confrontation with doctors. Many of the women thus served were not well-off and some had little prenatal care, yet the birth mortality reported by the nursing organisations that did this work was consistently less than half the birth mortality of the general population. This fact, although noted by medical officers of health and by the women's magazines from year to year, did not lead to any serious discussion of the possibility of legal midwifery in Canada until after the publication of a series of birth mortality inventories that shook obstetrics on both sides of the Atlantic.

The first of these publications, in 1929, gave the results of a ten-year maternal death survey from Aberdeen in Scotland. One disturbing fact stood out, described in the *Canadian Medical Association Journal* of 1929. 'The death rate per 1,000 maternity cases delivered by midwives was 2.8, by doctors 6.9 and in institutions 14.9. The last figure, which includes only cases untouched before admission, is surprisingly high.'[20] In Canada hospital birth mortality was also very much higher than that of birth at home,[21] although birth unattended by a physician was no longer separated as a category in our vital statistics and so its results were unknown.

The Aberdeen study received a good deal of attention in the Canadian medical press and resulted in the suggestion, by a few leading obstetricians, that legal midwifery should be introduced into Canada. Their case was strengthened by two major American reports, published in 1933, which concluded that two-thirds of maternal deaths could have been prevented had the doctors applied the best medical knowledge. The reports emphasised that despite the increase in hospital delivery, prenatal care, and aseptic technique, maternal mortality had not declined between 1915 and 1930. What was more, the number of infant deaths from birth injuries had *increased* by 40 to 50 per cent from 1915 to 1929.[22]

It appears from Canadian medical journals that physicians, particularly in Ontario and Quebec, took these American studies to be equally applicable in Canada. And when they looked at the countries that had the lowest maternal mortality rates – Holland, Denmark, Sweden, Norway and Italy (all less than half of Canada's rate) – it was undeniable that they all had at least one thing in common: their extensive use of midwives.

Suggestions appeared in the *Canadian Medical Association Journal* that perhaps it was time to send someone to those countries to examine their system. It is clear from the tone of these suggestions that their authors did not regard midwives, or the birth culture from which they came, as having useful kinds of knowledge in a positive sense. These obstetricians were concerned about the epidemic of obstetrical interventions that had overtaken the medical birth culture both in Europe and in North America, and they looked to midwives as persons who did not possess the tools that could damage mothers. It was not what midwives did do, but what they couldn't do, that made them interesting to obstetricians. This sentiment is evident in the correspondence between two physicians, one a leading obstetrician and one a government health official, soon after the release of the American maternal mortality reports:

> I know that there is a great antipathy to [the introduction of the midwife] on the part of my profession; but I have long felt that it is better for the average woman to be confined by someone who perforce cannot use more rigorous methods of getting a passenger through the pubic strait, than by a practitioner who is permitted, and often too willing, in order to save himself time, to use everything in his armamentarium, whether it's indicated or not. Then again, I think every obstetrical teacher in the country will agree that, considering what is expected of him in practice, the average medical graduate is woefully undertrained in obstetrics.[23]

In such an analysis, there were two solutions. Damage by doctors could be limited by taking the retrograde step of reintroducing the midwife, or by improving obstetrical teaching and obstetrical procedures already in use. The second step was more attractive to physicians, and after this time obstetrical teaching was expanded in Canadian medical schools.

As the shock and self-doubt initially produced by the Aberdeen, New York and White House studies wore off, there was a shift of attention from the doctors back to the birthing woman and her family. Hospitals, in an effort to reduce their mortality rates from puerperal fever, imposed more stringent controls on their maternity patients. Labouring women were strictly isolated from their non-medical family and friends, and medical personnel, particularly nurses, redoubled their efforts to degerm the woman and her environment. 'Medically unnecessary' approaches to the labouring woman were discouraged, and procedures as simple as an examination to check dilation were preceded by surgical antisepsis. This meant not only rigorous cleansing of the examiner but also shaving, douching, swabbing and purging of the woman herself. The labouring woman was instructed strictly to keep her hands away from the lower part of her body and to wear a mask if she had a cold, lest she transfer her mouth germs to her vagina and thus be the agent of her own demise. To ensure that she could not spoil the germ-free area so carefully set up around the lower part of her body, the woman's wrists were tied down during the latter part of her labour.

While professional midwifery made little headway in Canada, the geography of the country was such that the informal, neighbour birth culture could not be eliminated completely while frontier areas still existed. *The Canadian Mother and Child* estimated that 20,000 mothers delivered their babies without medical attendance in 1943, and 16,000 in 1947. Presuming these to be women in medically unserviced areas who relied on neighbours from necessity rather than choice, the author of *The Canadian Mother and Child*, Dr Ernest Couture, had made the decision to include a chapter on birth without a doctor in the 1940 edition so that the neighbour women might use the book as a resource. For this he was strongly criticised by Charlotte Whitton, head of the Child and Maternal Welfare Council in Ottawa:

> We must raise the question whether there might not be a danger . . . of this [chapter] being used by practical nurses and midwives to increase independence of the medical profession amongst certain ranks of the population, particularly among those of foreign birth.[24]

Dr Couture defended himself by saying that he was only trying to provide aid in a very undesirable situation, and that in his experience no mother would voluntarily have a baby without a doctor. Whether this was entirely true is questionable, especially since the 1947 edition begins with a reminder to women that doctors are more important than is generally acknowledged:

> A common opinion is that it is unnecessary to see a doctor, and this is based on the fallacy that, in the past, results were equally satisfactory when a doctor had not been consulted for pregnancy or even for childbirth.[25]

The majority of Canadian women had by that time been persuaded that unmedical birth was indeed a fallacy. But at the margins of settlement the traditional birth culture continued. The continuation of high maternal mortality statistics in hospitals and informal midwifery practised both by nurses and by neighbours in sparsely settled areas kept the issue of legal midwifery alive until well into the 1930s. Around 1937, there was a dramatic fall in maternal mortality in Europe and North America. This fall was particularly pronounced as it applied to mortality from puerperal infection, and it was evident in countries which continued to have domiciliary midwifery as well as those moving in the direction of universal hospital birth. Although the mortality rate began its dramatic decline a year before the introduction of the first antibiotic, in Canada it has usually been attributed to the considerable increase in hospital birth and the introduction of antibiotics. The attempt to link decreased morbidity and mortality with medical actions on a cause and effect basis is widespread, beyond the boundaries of obstetrics, but is being increasingly thrown into doubt by epidemiologists and statisticians. And indeed, when the fall in maternal mortality first became evident in Canada, some contemporary observers admitted to being mystified by it. In 1940, Dr A.H. Sellers, the Chief Statistician of the Dominion Bureau of Statistics, reported that while maternal mortality was the lowest since the collection of statistics had begun in 1920, 'no special change occurred during 1937–38, either in policy or in practice, which would appear to account for the improvement.'[26] A leading Canadian obstetrician, Dr B.P. Watson, then the head of a large maternity hospital in New York, admitted in 1938 that he had not yet had an opportunity to use the new drug 'prontosil' [sulfonamide],

> for it so happens that we have not had a single case of infection with a Group A beta haemolytic streptococcus since the drug came on the market. We do not flatter ourselves that this is due entirely to the precautions we take against its entry into our patients; other factors probably play a large part, the most important of which may be the epidemiological one. . . . It would appear that this is not a 'streptococcal year' in New York for I learn from my colleagues in other hospitals that their incidence of infections is also low.[27]

The independence of the introduction of antibiotics and the decline in maternal mortality due to sepsis was also evident in Britain:

> Prontosil was certainly not available for general use before 1937, by which year the number of (maternal) deaths from sepsis had fallen from 800 (1934) to half that figure – 347. Penicillin, similarly, was not available in Great Britain before 1946, by which year the number of deaths from sepsis had dropped to a mere 53 per annum.[28]

But while statisticians and some obstetricians might have been mystified by the fall in maternity mortality, the majority of medical workers were only too glad to announce that their labours had finally borne fruit, and that universal medicalised birth had brought obstetrics the dazzling success which it deserved. In Canada, hospital birth mortality fell to the level at which home birth mortality had stayed since the beginning of the Dominion Bureau of Statistics data collection, and then sank even lower. Home birth mortality slowly began to rise a little more every year as home birth became more and more rare, and more confined to accidents, premature birth, and to endangered economic groups such as Canada's native people. Any talk of midwives as safer practitioners stopped.

This is not to say that midwifery stopped, or that the popular birth culture died out altogether. In Newfoundland, in Labrador, and in areas of the north that were still attracting new settlers, as well as in rural pockets here and there throughout the country, neighbours continued to help one another at times of childbirth. But in all these places there was increasingly a consciousness that unmedical birth was on its way out, that it was a stop-gap until there were sufficient hospitals and doctors to enable all births to be conducted 'properly'.

There was, however, one large area of Canada where the notion came later that unmedical birth was unnatural. Before the 1960s, there were very few medical births among those native Indian or Inuit peoples who lived in the northern part of the provinces and in the North-west Territories. Although most native communities seem to have had a number of women recognised as midwives, the seasonal migrations of the largely hunter-gatherer societies meant birth knowledge had to be wide-spread in the community. The native birth culture was therefore similar to the neighbourly birth culture as it had developed among the European settlers in the previous century. Non-native medical workers who had contact with native communities after the 1950s were impressed by the level of skill among those women whom they saw helping out at births. Retained placenta, breech births, and haemorrhage were all difficulties which seem to have been within the ability of the midwives to handle. Disproportion seems to have been very rare, perhaps because full-term native babies tended to be small. Labours among native women, when not complicated by serious diseases such as active tuberculosis, or by malnutrition, were in general very efficient and short.

The large-scale involvement of medical workers with the native birth culture came about as the result of a campaign by the Canadian government, beginning in the 1950s, to increase its staff of northern nurses and physicians in an effort to do battle with tuberculosis there. Once the nurses and doctors were in the north, the original objective was expanded to include the delivery of all types of modern medical service, including medical childbirth. The very high mortality rate which accompanied the marginal economic condition of the Indian and Inuit people was redefined as a medical problem, for which white medical workers would provide the solutions.

Moving childbirth out of the tents and igloos was a gradual process, limited both by the cost of increasing medical facilities and by the reluctance of native people to abandon their birth culture. There was also some ambivalence on the part of the government medical workers about the usefulness of the project. Dr Otto Schaefer, for example, who began with the Medical Services Branch in 1952, recalls that at the beginning he was not convinced of the need for more hospital deliveries, and deliveries in nursing stations, because in his experience the number of complications in hunting camp deliveries, still handled by the native midwives, seemed to be no higher than in the births handled by the nurses.[29] There were only very limited attempts to evaluate mortality and morbidity data prior to the implementation of the new policy, however, since it was regarded as axiomatic that any move in the direction of medicalized birth would be a move toward better health.

The nurses who came to work in the north began at once to persuade the local women to have their babies at nursing stations. They also offered a package of prenatal care which included the no-cost provision of vitamins and food supplements to needy mothers. It seemed that the white government was beginning to make good its long-standing promise of providing the same services to native people as those which it made available to the non-native women in the south.

In fact, native women were receiving a service which it had not been possible to get for the south. Beginning in the 1960s, the Canadian government actively recruited midwives in Great Britain, Australia and New Zealand to work in northern Canada. There was no medical opposition to this policy because it was understood that the service dealt exclusively with native women. From the very beginning, the few white women living in the north were flown out to a southern hospital for childbirth, whereas the government midwives delivered the native women in the northern nursing stations, unless they were judged at special risk.

Many of the government midwives worked hard to accommodate themselves to the local birth culture, and relations between them and the traditional birth helpers were often friendly. Some midwives took special care to ensure that traditional birth attendants continued to be present at births in the nursing stations, so that the kinship relationships originating from birth attendance would not be so disrupted. In a situation where little dramatic action could be taken if problems arose, the midwives altered their practice to include less auscultation of the foetal heart and more simple support for the mother. In practice many of their activities during childbirth were not so very different from those traditional to the native birth culture.

About fifteen years after the first government midwives came into the native communities, there began to be a gradual shift in government policy in favour of reducing the number of local births in nursing stations and evacuating a larger number of native women to distant hospitals for childbirth. This shift in policy was based not on an evaluation of mortality data[30] but on the belief of government policy makers in the superior safety of hospital births. Initially only primiparas and grand multiparas were added to the evacuation lists, but by the end of the 1970s, the official goal became 100 per cent maternal evacuation. A number of factors contributed to hastening this process. Immigration laws were tightened and it became more difficult to bring foreign midwives into the country. Canadian nurses, even when given a special four-month course to prepare them for their northern duties, lacked the confidence that they could handle births. The system of supportive obstetricians available for telephone consultations and regular doctor visits to nursing stations crumbled. Mary Stevenson, an Irish midwife formerly working in Labrador, observed that as the policy of total evacuation became more pronounced, the nurses became more nervous about doing low-risk deliveries, even when their results were excellent. Stevenson felt that there came to be an atmosphere of crisis around birth.[31] Many of the nurses were young and inexperienced (the average age in nursing stations in northern Ontario was 22; the average stay in many areas was less than one year). They were less willing than the foreign-trained midwives had been to be on call twenty-four hours a day and to work the extra hours required of them when there was a maternity patient at the station. If a mother did go into labour before she could be sent out, it was not uncommon for the nurse to send her to hospital, together with her baby, on the next flight out, so that postpartum care could be handled elsewhere.

The reduction in births at the nursing stations also resulted in a real decline in the competence of the nurses, since they now had very little chance to deliver babies. In many ways, then, the policy of considering birth as too dangerous to be handled by midwives outside hospital became a self-fulfilling prophecy.

Canada's ambitious attempt to install a safe midwifery system across the north has now crumbled into remnants. Reaction from the native population has been varied, ranging from acceptance, to specific complaints about hospital procedures, to a more general rejection of evacuation. That rejection seems to be most pronounced among Inuit people, and is apparently leading some Inuit women to once again avoid prenatal care, and in some extreme situations to run and hide when the plane comes to fly them out. Evacuation has become an important political issue in some communities, where the tribal councils assert that the removal of all births from the communities constitutes a major assault on their cultural integrity. If the determination to avoid evacuation spreads, it is unclear how the government can respond. One of the reasons for the dismantling of the nursing-station births was the difficulty of finding nurse-midwives who would wish to work so far from home, and would stay there long enough to build up a relationship with the local people. Some native groups are calling for a return to the local midwife, who is part of the community and will not leave after half a year. As one tribal elder asserts, 'The people are fighting back. They're saying, "We've done it for generations and we can do it ourselves." But if we wait much longer, the people will forget how to do it, and it will be too late.'[32] There are indeed still older women in many native communities who can remember participating in births before the government medical workers became involved. But over a period of almost thirty years, the government nurses and nurse-midwives spread the message as part of their public health work that the local birth culture was inferior to the medical birth culture. Although some nurse-midwives tried to make an accommodation with the traditional birth culture, there was never an attempt to keep the local midwives practising, on any terms. There are now some non-native health workers who also believe that native midwifery must return. However, reconstituting the original culture from the fragments that remain is bound to be very difficult. Nonetheless, in a few northern communities a consensus about the importance of the manner of birth is once again growing among the different generations. In the Keewatin area of the North-west Territories, the determination of the tribal councils to reintegrate births into their communities has gained considerable media coverage nationwide. There are also a few instances, recently, of white medical workers attempting to draw native women back into practice. In Povungnituk, near Hudson's Bay, the maternity 'team' of the local hospital consists of several non-Inuit doctors, two non-Inuit nurse-midwives and five Inuit birth assistants who attend births and also take part in all treatment decision meetings, where they have, formally at least, influence equal to the medically trained members of the team.

The experiment in Povungnituk was conceived by a nurse-midwife from southern Quebec, who was herself a participant in a revival of the popular birth culture that began in many different areas across Canada in the early 1970s. Some traditional religious families, especially among orthodox Jews, Roman Catholics, and Jehovah's Witnesses, had continued to have their babies at home without fanfare throughout the 1950s and 1960s, either on their own or with the help of a few physicians who had never stopped delivering babies at home. These families felt that hospital birth secularised and threw away the powerful meaning of the birth event. When the 1970s brought a rising interest on the part of many people in simplifying their lives and avoiding institutions, the number of births outside hospital began to increase. In a few cities there were doctors who accommodated themselves to this new trend, but in most places medicine denounced or ridiculed birth at home. It came about, then, that pregnant women and their partners and friends had to reinvent a birth culture for themselves. In some ways doctors were just as absent for them as they were for the early settlers when they first arrived from Europe.

This birth culture as it developed during the 1970s was very diverse. It accommodated orthodox religious groups, members of recently imported eastern religions, members of various parts of the counter-culture, and a considerable number of fairly mainstream middle-class women who were simply unwilling to subject themselves to hospital birth. Feminism was an important element in many of the groups. Birth styles varied and reflected the needs and capacities of a wide variety of families. As in the birth culture evolved by the original settlers in the nineteenth century, mortality and morbidity were only sketchily documented, but there is likewise evidence that birth outcome was on the whole very satisfactory.

Because of the long hiatus in non-medical birth, manuals detailing the natural stages of labour and birth substituted for the helpful neighbour woman at the beginning. As more women gained experience in giving birth under normal circumstances, they began attending births of friends and helping one another. While some of the subgroups of the birth culture continued to restrict birth attendance to their own intimate circle, there came to be a demand for midwives from other families.

At the beginning very few of the women who offered themselves as midwives were formally trained to do this work. While they augmented their experience with weekend workshops, observation and labour coaching in hospitals, and occasionally short courses taken outside the country, the style of practice of most of these midwives was very informal. Many of their clients were or became their friends. Payment, if any, was worked out on the ability to pay and sometimes took the form of barter. Prenatal visits were usually informal and took place at irregular intervals. At the births, there were often other friends attending, with the midwife only one player in the event. Midwives not only supported the mother but also helped care for other children, or prepared food, or cleaned up during and after the birth.

As the midwives began to accumulate experience, apprenticeship became the most common point of entry for new midwives. The need for a somewhat more predictable schedule to accommodate apprentices was one factor which led some midwives to establish 'clinic' times with appointments and set procedures similar to those carried out at the prenatal clinics run by doctors. Another reason for the more formal clinics was that midwives began to have an increased client load. This was partly because of the wide and often enthusiastic media attention given to home birth, making more people aware of this possibility, and partly because some midwives began to actively seek more clients, as they found that increased public acceptance of birth alternatives made midwifery a viable career.

The new legitimacy given to midwives had its problems. For one thing, it made them a more obvious irritation to the medical profession, which was potentially able to express its displeasure, since midwifery was not legal in most provinces of Canada. Just as importantly, as their clientele increased, the connection between client and midwife became more tenuous. This meant that the midwife could make fewer assumptions about the culture and outlook of her clients and also that the client's expectations of the midwives might be shaped not by stories heard from friends but by an idealised public image of the midwife, which the midwife then needed to live up to.

The work of the midwife began to be altered by some of the same pressures found in orthodox medical practice. Issues of thorough documentation in case of litigation, uniform standards, group practice to preserve free time and privacy, and conformity to association norms came more to the foreground.

Around the time when midwives began to see themselves as a new kind of health worker, the influence of feminists who had experience in political work began to grow stronger within the alternative birth culture. The birth culture, previously diverse and highly anarchic, underwent a shift as leaders emerged. There began to be much discussion about goals and strategies, and a new focus on the role of the midwife as the central player in the birth culture. Several ambitious conferences, which included midwives from other parts of the world, strengthened the intention of birth activists to work for legal status for the midwife, so that she would begin to take the honoured position within the maternity care system that she deserved. Midwifery task forces, composed either entirely of lay members or of a combination of lay and medical representatives, were formed in Montreal, Toronto and Vancouver. Although their original position was that midwifery must be legalised in order to respond to the clear desire by certain women to be cared for by a midwife, in some areas their goals broadened to financing midwives through health insurance and giving an opportunity to all women to benefit from a midwife-conducted birth.

Political lobbying and extensive use of the media by activists within the birth culture resulted in the opening of midwifery demonstration projects in hospitals in Vancouver and in Hamilton, Ontario, and in the announcement, in 1985, that the government of Ontario was setting up its own task force to establish how midwifery could be integrated into maternity care in that province. Although these developments were greeted with enthusiasm by many birth activists, this reaction was not shared by everyone. Some women and men who had been involved in the alternative birth culture from the beginning reacted with dismay as midwives appeared to be moving closer to professionalisation. Negative reaction was and is strongest among those who had originally recommended decriminalisation of midwifery rather than licensing, on the grounds that licensing midwives would simply establish a new monopoly. The dismay expressed by this group increased as pressure mounted on the new almost-legal midwives not to deviate from fairly conservative standards of safe practice at home births. While most midwives still atttended births of first-time mothers at home even though this practice had been declared unsafe by the medical orthodoxy, births of twins, births with a previous difficult obstetrical history, births with the baby in breech position, and particularly vaginal births after caesareans, are now refused by most midwives. Since the percentage of caesarean operations has risen to the level of an epidemic in many parts of this country, the last category in particular includes a quickly rising number of women, some of whom feel passionately that hospitals are dangerous for them. In a remarkable turn of the wheel there are now women who once again give birth unattended by any experienced woman, because they refuse to leave their homes to have their babies, no matter where they have been ranked on a medical risk scoring form.

Some midwives have attempted to deal with the gap between obstetric risk scoring and client demands by introducing the newly current language of ethics into their practice. They assert that it is the ethical responsibility of a midwife to follow the wishes of the mother, even a high-risk mother who has refused to budge from her choice of a home birth. This language enables the midwife to circumvent the medical accusation that midwives are women who engage in practices that have been declared marginal or dangerous by mainstream obstetrics. Instead, the midwife is behaving in a highly ethical manner if she lays out all the medical information she possesses to explain the risks to her client, but still accepts the final decision of the mother. Whether such a structuring of birth really ends up with the mother feeling that she is free to do as she wishes is in question. A way in which one group of midwives has dealt with the refusal of clients to go to hospital is by summoning an ambulance to the house. If the client turns the ambulance attendants away, there is then an official record that the midwife was not responsible for the client's decision. One wonders what effect such a scenario has on the alternative birth culture.

There is no doubt that the midwife's need to protect herself from possible medical retribution has influenced her practice, especially in the last five or six years as she has become a potentially serious competitor with the doctor for maternity clients. Whether legalisation will give the midwife the security she needs to develop into a truly alternative maternity care worker or whether, instead, continued compromises with the obstetric establishment will turn her into the Trojan Horse of the alternative birth culture, remains to be seen.

NOTES

1   Audrey Saunders Miller (ed.), *The Journals of Mary O'Brien, 1828–1838*, Macmillan, 1968, p. 231.
2   Ibid., p. 234.
3   Clara Ann Tarrant, Newfoundland midwife, interviewed for Canadian Broadcasting Corporation, CBC Radio, 1979, CBC Tape Archives, nos. 750514–18.
4   Mrs Lillian Miles, Edenwold, Saskatchewan, Saskatchewan Archives Board, Pioneer Questionnaires (Health) SX–2.
5   H. Gordon Green, *Don't Have Your Baby in the Dory: A Biography of Myra Bennett*, Harvest House, 1974.
6   Jo Lutley, nurse-midwife, interviewed for 'Doctoring the family', Canadian Broadcasting Corporation, CBC Radio, *Ideas* series, prepared by David Cayley and Jutta Mason, broadcast on CBC 4–25 April 1985, transcript published by CBC Transcripts, Montreal, 1985.
7   W.A. Bigelow, *Forceps, Fin and Feather: Memoirs of Dr W.A. Bigelow*, D.W. Friesen & Sons, 1969.
8   M. Seymour, MD, cited by Leslie Biggs in 'The response to maternal mortality in Ontario, 1920–1940', unpublished master's thesis, University of Toronto, 1983, p. 113.
9   E.W. Montgomery, Minister of Health for Manitoba, 'Maternal mortality', *Canadian Public Health Journal*, vol. 21, 1930, p. 219.
10 From Red Cross Archives File, Red Cross House, Toronto. Correspondence between Mrs C.B. Waagen, Honorary Secretary of the Committee on Policy, and Dr Fred Routley, Director of the Ontario Division of the Red Cross.
11 Leslie Biggs, 'The case of the missing midwives: a history of midwifery in Ontario, 1795–1900', *Ontario History*, vol. 75, no. 1, 1983, pp. 21–35. See also *The Hamilton Times*, 17 July 1915 and *Report of the Task Force for the Implementation of Midwifery in Ontario*, Appendix 1.
12 Benjamin Atlee, MD, taped interview by sociologist Kathy Moggridge, Halifax, 1978.
13 Public Archives of Canada, *The Victorian Order of Nurses*, MG. 27, 1 B5, vol. 10, 'Memorandum to Montreal Local Council of Women', 1897.
14 John Campbell Gordon, First Marquis of Aberdeen and Temair, *We Twa: Reminiscences of Lord and Lady Aberdeen*, vol. 2, Collins, 1926, p. 121.
15 Helen MacMurchy, MD, *Maternal Mortality in Canada: Report of an Enquiry Made by the Department of Health*, Dept of Health Canada, Ottawa, 1928.

16   Linda Rasmussen, Lorna Rasmussen, Candace Savage and Anne Wheeler, *A Harvest Yet to Reap: A History of Prairie Women*, The Women's Press, 1976, p. 76.

17   Helen MacMurchy, MD, *The Canadian Mother's Book*, Dept of Health, Ottawa, 1927, publication no. 2 of Confederation Diamond Jubilee edition, p. 24.

18   Public Archives of Canada, *Maternal and Child Welfare Department*, vol. 992, file 499–3–7, Roy Dafoe, MD, *A Country Doctor Speaks to Women*.

19   Public Archives of Canada, *Department of Health*, RG. vol. 991, file 499–3–2 (part 3). Letter from Mrs Leonard Renaud, Wawbewawa, Ontario, to the Department of Health, Ottawa, 10 July 1935.

20   A.D. Blackader, 'Thoughts on maternal mortality', *Canadian Medical Association Journal*, June 1929, p. 656.

21   *Report of the Task Force for the Implementation of Midwifery in Ontario*, Appendix 1.

22   New York Academy of Medicine, *Maternal Mortality in New York City*, New York, Commonwealth Fund, 1933. See also White House Conference on Child Health and Protection Study, cited by Richard W. Wertz and Dorothy C. Wertz in *Lying-In – A History of Childbirth in America*, Schocken Books, 1979.

23   Public Archives of Canada, *Maternal and Child Welfare Department*, vol. 992, file 499–3–7, part 6.

24   Public Archives of Canada, *Maternal and Child Welfare Department*, vol. 992, file 499–3–7, part 6. Letter from Charlotte Whitton to Ernest Couture, 5 October 1940.

25   Ernest Couture, *The Canadian Mother and Child*, Seventh Printing, King's Printer, 1947.

26   A.H. Sellers, MD, 'Vital statistics: the recent improvement in maternal mortality in Canada', *Canadian Public Health Journal*, vol. 31, 1940, p. 38.

27   B.P. Watson, 'Puerperal sepsis', *Canadian Medical Association Journal*. February 1938, pp. 139–42.

28   A.J. Wrigley, 'Observations on maternal mortality', in R.J. Kellar (ed.), *Modern Trends in Obstetrics*, vol. 3, Butterworths, 1963.

29   Dr Otto Schaefer, interviewed in October 1986, cited in Appendix 1, *Report of the Task Force on the Implementation of Midwifery in Ontario*, op. cit.

30   In fact, the few mortality data that exist suggest that when more women were evacuated, birth mortality did not diminish significantly. T.F. Baskett, 'Obstetric care in the central Canadian Arctic', *British Medical Journal*, vol. 2, 1978, pp. 1002–4; T.F. Baskett *et al.*, 'Obstetrical emergencies in the Canadian Arctic', *Proceedings of the International Conference on Circumpolar Health*,

Nordic Council, Copenhagen, 1981.

31 Mary Stevenson, Lecturer in Outpost Nursing, Dalhousie University School of Nursing, Halifax, cited in Appendix 1, *Report of the Task Force on the Implementation of Midwifery in Ontario*, op. cit.

32 *The Globe and Mail*, 10 November 1986. Also 'Inuit fight loneliness for safe births', *Toronto Star*, 23 March 1987.

INTRODUCTION

BANGLADESH AND GUATEMALA

In many Third World countries women are the silent half of the adult population. When they will not be silent, they are silenced.

Traditionally health care has been in the hands of women and all over the world it has taken place in domestic territory controlled by women. As countries become westernised health care is appropriated by men, removed from the home, and professionalised. As a result, patterns of care which are integrated with that specific culture break down. The traditional herbal pharmacopoeia, women's empirical knowledge about the treatment of illness, and rituals providing emotional support and comfort to individuals and families in the life crises of birth and death, are forgotten. Midwifery skills are no longer handed down from older to younger women, from mothers to daughters, and in the absence of care women have to cope as best they can. Those who can afford to do so go to doctors, and the North American model of childbirth becomes the norm.

Yet the indigenous midwife has many advantages. She belongs to the local community. She knows and is in regular contact with the women she attends and their families. She is on the spot and speedily available. She understands, and often shares, the poverty in which they live, and the social pressures they are under. Her beliefs about health and illness, pregnancy, birth and babies are the same as those of the women she serves.

She works under conditions which might be intolerable to any trained midwife – not only without modern drugs and equipment, but in places where every drop of water is precious, where it has to be brought from the nearest accessible stream or well by women bowed like beasts of burden, and where the only method of boiling water is slow and laborious. She delivers babies in hovels where animals share the dwelling, often in semi-darkness, and with the ever-present risk of a thatched roof catching light from an open fire.

When a medical system is superimposed from outside, the indigenous midwife loses whatever status she had in her community. Women are warned against using her on the grounds that she is dirty and illiterate, and does not know how to deal with complications. If she sends a mother to hospital because labour is protracted, the placenta is retained, or there is haemorrhage, the authorities notch it up as another example of the danger of folk midwives, and harangue the mother and family members for seeking her help. Thus she is discouraged from making referrals to hospital – and the split between the indigenous and official health care systems becomes wider still.

The benefits of the new technology need to be weighed against the hazards of obstetric intervention and invasive procedures which may prove harmful for mothers and babies. In Yucatan the traditional method of treating the newborn baby's umbilical cord is to cut it with a fresh slice of bamboo and then to slowly and carefully cauterise the stump in a candle flame.[1] Now indigenous midwives are instructed to cut it with scissors and to use alcohol and an antiseptic. But in a hut without boiling water it is impossible to sterilise scissors properly and dabbing on alcohol is less effective than burning the stump.

An important characteristic of low technology is that it is simple and easily obtained, interchanged and replaced. It is enmeshed in the cultural matrix. Yet it is much easier to transport the high technology, and the procedures which go along with it, than this low technology that is anchored in culture. In Africa, for example, a woman may hold a rope slung from the rafters during labour, but no one is going to transport ropes from Africa so that women in the west can do the same. There is no fortune to be made out of selling ropes.[2] In many countries attempts are being made to incorporate indigenous midwives and other healers into the official system. But such efforts have often been frustrated by prejudice against them on the part of trained staff. In the Caribbean, for example, when in the 1960s *nanas* were given short courses on basic cleanliness, aseptic technique, accurate weighing of babies, and complications of pregnancy and birth which should result in referral to hospital, the initiative broke down because of organised opposition from doctors, midwives and nurses who felt their own status threatened by the recognition of *nanas*. Yet in spite of this opposition from the medical system the World Health Organisation, recognising that 70 per cent of babies in many parts of the world are delivered by 'traditional birth attendants', supports their training and encourages policies which incorporate them into health care systems.

Another major problem with the introduction of high-tech obstetrics in these societies is that it is, for the most part, inappropriate to the needs of local people and inaccessible to the vast majority. It may be available to those who live within the catchment areas of large hospitals and regional centres, but women in rural areas have no access to it. Obstetric high technology, however, is eagerly received by the governments of developing countries, where the hospitals in which it is enthroned consume a disproportionate amount of the health care budget. In Senegal and Tanzania, for example, high-tech hospitals absorb more than half of the total budget available for health care, while serving only 5 per cent of the population.[3]

In many developing countries midwifery has become a bad word. Midwives are synonymous with ancient, discarded and despised traditions, and with ignorance and poverty. When this happens, professional midwives find that the way is barred to them also. Only doctors have high status, and high-tech obstetrics is seen as guaranteeing safety.

The introduction of high technology always has profound effects on the social system. Oxfam has pointed out that in agriculture, development projects have benefited men, but have led to a reduction in women's status and a narrowing of the range of options open to women.[4] In childbirth, high technology is associated with a hierarchical system of power and decision-making, since the information necessary to make decisions is embedded in the technology itself, and only experts control it. When low technology is available, decisions about the right course of action are made by everyone involved in the process of childbirth.

The next two chapters focus on societies in parts of the world which are geographically far apart and culturally distinct, but which share many of the problems of poverty, disruptive social change that holds both threat and promise, and the exploitation and subjugation of women.

NOTES

1 Brigitte Jordan, 'High technology: the case of obstetrics', *World Health Forum*, vol. 8, 1987, pp. 312–38.

2 Ibid.
3 Ibid.
4 B. Pratt and J. Boyden (eds), *The Field Directors' Handbook: An Oxfam Manual for Development Workers*, Oxford University Press, 1985.

THE BIRTH ATTENDANT IN BANGLADESH

FRANCES McCONVILLE

In Bangladesh, the third poorest country in the world with a population of approximately 110 million, only 1 to 2 per cent of women deliver their babies in health facilities with trained personnel present. It is distressing, though not surprising, that the maternal mortality rate is estimated to be six per 1,000, or a hundred times that of developed countries. Approximately one in five infants die, many from causes directly related to childbirth.

There are no institutionalised 'midwives', no stereotypical 'traditional birth attendants' working their way around the villages. Many Moslem women deliver on their own, but most deliver with the assistance of female relatives, or *dais*. Few women in critical condition reach the help of the handful of doctors who, along with the nurse-midwives, are doing their best to combine an archaic British training with their status as Moslem women. These women are brought together under conditions that evoke Florence Nightingale's descriptions of the Crimea. Yet at the same time, for the Islamic women birth is the ultimate identifying experience. For the first time in her life motherhood will bring to her at least some status as a woman. Paradoxically, the joyous event is shrouded in mystery, and she must be humiliated by her shame. In a society where women are valued for little other than their fertility, the need for the birth of a healthy child is paramount.

The birth attendants today are thus facing a difficult situation. Disparate, poorly trained, ill-equipped, socially segregated and politically powerless, they strive to meet the fundamental need for the future of their society, safe delivery.

THE ORIGINS OF THE PRESENT-DAY BIRTH ATTENDANT

As in many Islamic areas of Asia, childbirth has for centuries been shrouded in the mystery of the women in 'purdah'. Birth rituals, and the traditional practices of the birth attendants, have been derived from the interpretation of experiences at births, and superstitious, religious and cultural beliefs. These complex interactions have been compounded by political events.

Traditional birth rituals

The greatest influence over the traditional birth rituals has been a combination of the Islamic religion and 'purdah', the associated concept of 'pollution', and the belief in evil spirits or *bhuts*. As with many religious or superstitious rituals, these beliefs stem from a strongly patriarchal system and deep-rooted fears of women's sexuality.

For the majority of women, illiterate, insulated from life outside the village and excluded from the mosque, the Moslem religion exerts a predominantly social influence. Obvious recognisable behaviours, such as the covering of the body in a *burka*, and restriction from travel and exposure, are aimed at protecting the honour of women.

Common to the Moslem and Hindu women, and associated with 'purdah', is the concept of 'pollution'. Women are said to be in a state of 'pollution' during menstruation, whilst pregnant, and in the postnatal period. This is because women's blood, stored and stagnant in the body for these functions, is believed to be impure, unlike the blood of a fresh wound. As a result, women in a polluted state bring shame upon themselves should they pollute others. In some cases women remain housebound during menstruation and are similarly restricted during pregnancy. The cutting of the umbilical cord is the most polluting act during delivery, and whoever attends the birth is implicated.

The evil spirits or *bhuts* further complicate these issues by being particularly attracted to the pregnant or breastfeeding woman, and to the child itself from conception until the cessation of breastfeeding. If the woman is to avoid angering the *bhuts* then she should, for example, keep her hair tied up tightly and not leave the home, or *bari*, at midday or dusk.

Who were the dais?

According to anthropologist Thérèse Blanchet, these factors determine who, if anyone, has traditionally attended a birth. For the Hindu woman the presence of a *dai* is essential because she performs the function of transferring the pollution upon herself. She will, for example, cut the umbilical cord, and thereby keeps the household in an unpolluted state. The Hindu *dai* originates from a low-caste family and may be paid for the job she has inherited.

The presence of a *dai* to remove pollution is not required for Moslem women, and to this day it is thought that up to a third of Moslem women, isolated in their personal shame, experience delivery on their own. Many, for the same reason, are reluctant to seek medical help when complications arise. Usually the husband's female relatives will attend the delivery (as the married woman lives with the husband's family), relatives being less easily polluted than neighbours. The Moslem *dai* may not, however, always cut the umbilical cord. Instead she may ask the mother to do it, or pay someone else a small fee. The Moslem *dai* does not usually receive payment, but may be given a gift, such as a sari.

Although the above distinctions were recorded by Thérèse Blanchet in her detailed study of a rural area, it is not clear that the pattern is rigid throughout the land. The area is culturally rich in its regional variations, and to many women childbirth has always been a powerful, but essentially private, experience.

Traditional practices of the dais

The traditional practices of the *dais* or attendant relatives continue to this day, and have been similarly influenced by 'purdah', 'pollution' and *bhuts*. Regional variations persist. Many practices are positive and many others are harmful.

Positive practices

The most attractive custom is that delivery has traditionally taken place in the home with the supportive company of other women friends or relatives. Pain relief in the form of drugs has never been available. Instead constant and close physical contact by means of massaging is provided, along with intense emotional support. Position at delivery is chosen by the woman to maximise pain relief (as opposed to convenience for the attender) and the kneeling position with the head and arms resting on the bed or a wooden *choki* is most favoured. Mobility is also encouraged. Where attendants are present, they will not leave the labouring woman until all is complete. In the days following delivery the baby is always kept close by the mother. Most families sleep together on the one large *choki*, and the responsibility for the baby is easily, and readily, shared. The mother is never left to cope on her own, and the baby receives a great deal of attention. The state of 'pollution' that continues up to forty days postnatally allows the mother time for recuperation. Breastfeeding has always been, naturally, at the baby's demand, and is continued for one, two, or even more years. Problems with breastfeeding are virtually unheard of.

Harmful practices
Notably, most harmful practices are influenced by what is seen as 'pollution', and appreciably logical approaches to reducing risks at delivery. Food restrictions, for example, are common practice in an attempt to prevent large babies and difficult deliveries. Protein-rich foods, in particular fish, mutton, duck, eggs and shrimps, are commonly withheld. In some regions one type of fish is thought to cause 'fits', and one particular variety of large fish is not eaten, as to cut it into pieces would anger the gods, who would then take revenge on the child. It is thought that the twisted and contorted shape of ginger (the basis of many curries) causes a child to be crippled, that pineapple induces abortion, and sweet pumpkin causes coughs. Eclamptic fits (all too frequent a phenomenon) are believed to be caused by the *bhuts*. Oedema is not recognised as a potential problem.

The combined forces of 'purdah' and *bhuts*, whilst protecting the pregnant woman, effectively restrict her mobility and prevent her from seeking help.

At the time of delivery, 'pollution', as opposed to asepsis, bears greatest influence. Birth itself is considered a dirty event, taking place on the earth floor or an old mat. The cleansing of the woman, her clothes, the environment and all equipment takes place after delivery, in order to wash away polluted blood. Some items such as the placenta or clothes are burnt or buried. In some Hindu areas a practice has been to build a special hut for delivery, which is destroyed after the forty postnatal days.

The left hand, associated with dirt and faeces, is used for vaginal examinations and perineal guarding. The birth attendant may also apply her foot to the perineum. Non-sterile lubricants, such as coconut or mustardseed oil, are used for frequent vaginal examinations, performed in attempts to expedite delivery. Once the membranes have been deliberately ruptured delivery is encouraged to take place, irrespective of cervical dilatation. Fundal pressure is often applied. In prolonged labour a tight band is tied around the abdomen to prevent the baby coming 'upwards'. An old rag may be placed on the baby's head to pull the body out. An old nail or rusty kitchen knife may be used for an episiotomy.

Expulsion of the placenta, the 'life force', is done quickly, as the newborn baby is not considered fully alive until this has happened. The placenta might be pulled out, abdominal pressure applied, or the cord repeatedly pricked. The woman's hair may be soaked in an oil such as kerosene and stuffed in her mouth to induce vomiting action which will hopefully push out the placenta. In some regions haemorrhaging is considered a good sign, ridding the body of polluted blood.

Care of the newborn is withheld until delivery of the placenta is complete. Until this has occurred, the baby is left cold and wet on the floor, no resuscitative measures being taken. Cutting of the umbilical cord is usually done with a bamboo sliver or old knife. To help dry out the umbilical stump, powdered cow dung, ash, or burning hot oil are applied.

Colostrum, believed to be 'bad milk', is withheld for three days. Replacement feeds such as honey and cow's milk, or mustard oil, diluted with warm pond or river water are given. Postnatally fluid and food restriction are continued. The mother is considered to be in a 'wet' state. Dry foods such as *muri* (puffed rice) are given, but many nutritious moist foods are withheld.

It is clear that harmful practices contribute to the present-day mortality and morbidity rates. The major causes of maternal death have been identified as infection, eclampsia, haemorrhage and other complications. Statistics are variable. The concept of 'pollution' is obviously related to the drastically high number of women who die from puerperal sepsis and tetanus. Eclampsia is frequent, largely due to endemic anaemia compounded by food restrictions and the belief in *bhuts*. Maternal malnutrition is now understood to be the cause of the 'low birth weight' syndrome. Death from postpartum haemorrhage is clearly associated with methods of expelling the placenta and, again, polluted blood. The major recorded causes of morbidity or mortality in infants have been recognised as tetanus, pneumonia, birth trauma and prematurity. It is thought, though not entirely understood, that women are reluctant to seek help partly because of 'purdah' and the *bhuts*, though many other factors prevail.

The influence of history

Changes in the role and identity of some of the birth attendants have gradually been brought about by the course of history, including the British Raj, the East Pakistan period, and in particular the recent emergence of modern–day Bangladesh.

The British Raj left behind in India a legacy of impenetrable bureaucracy, along with laudable public services, including hospitals, and the establishment of British-style schools of medicine, nursing and midwifery. Unfortunately little thought was given to the cultural as opposed to the medical needs of the childbearing woman or her birth attendant. To this day only 1 to 2 per cent of deliveries take place in hospitals, where separation of a woman from her home and family, at so crucial a time, is not acceptable. In addition the change from the physical and emotional support given to women by the *dais* to control by unfamiliar, and often male, obstetricians or medical students seems only to have intensified the humiliation and shame associated with 'purdah', and inadvertently to have reinforced women's trust in one another.

To the uneducated *dai* the presence of hospitals brought little change. For other Moslem and Hindu women, however, the formal western style of nursing and midwifery created problems. Not only were the obstetric practices or management of complications of little relevance to East Bengal, but the birth attendant's role as 'midwife' had little similarity to that of her European contemporaries, and to this day social mores, amongst other factors, prevent the so-called 'midwife' from practising fully as a professional birth attendant. In reality, another vague administrative level was introduced. The training of women obstetricians was a most positive step, although again they are limited to work in city hospitals.

Despite the turmoil of the period 1947–71, when Bangladesh was known as East Pakistan, the government of this time introduced the concept of 'primary health care'. Within the new infrastructure, and reflecting the more appropriate approach, was a new cadre of women health workers, the 'lady health visitors'. This was a village-based job following twenty-one months of a training programme that gave some emphasis to delivery.

The devastating civil war that established independent Bangladesh in 1971, and the concurrent floods and famines, resulted in massive international relief work. Subsequently development agencies have become entrenched, but with no noticeable effect on the survival rates of women and children, nor on the role of the birth attendants. The lady health visitor has been replaced by the less well trained family welfare visitor (FWV). The UNICEF-supported Government Traditional Birth Attendant Training Programme was hampered by administrative setbacks, and midwifery training has yet to be upgraded. Great emphasis has been given to 'population control', in contrast to the low profile maintained for the actual health of women and children. The late 1980s have however seen a potential popularisation of the issue of maternal health, and with the backing of the UN agencies the government has recognised 'safe delivery' as one of its top priorities.

THE PRESENT-DAY BIRTH ATTENDANT

The situation remains that 'midwives', as a professional coordinated group, do not exist. There is, instead, a socially divided and disparate workforce. These women are potentially united by their desire to provide care for other women, despite abysmal pay and conditions. They are exceptional in that they are prepared to overcome traditional opposition in order to go out and work. The birth attendants are, perhaps unknowingly, in a unique position. Apart from motherhood itself there is no greater nor more acceptable link between women than the job of assisting in childbirth. The persisting mortality and morbidity rates are indicative of the overwhelming need to develop this as yet untapped, but dynamic, resource. The hierarchy of birth attendants is as follows: doctors, nurse-midwives, family welfare visitors (FWVs), trained 'traditional birth attendants' (TBAs), and then the *dais*, relatives of the woman herself. The order is absolutely determined by the strong cultural forces that prevail and there is no manoeuvring up or down the strata. Given the social patterns of the Bangladeshi (Islamic) culture, it is uncommon for relationships, professional or personal, to develop between women of different social status. Barriers to communication result from poverty, lack of education and variations in dialect, and are reinforced by the complex roles of the women in the home. The professional woman of the 1980s, a doctor for example, is, to some extent, independent of these traditions, but remains closely within the family unit. To live, work, or even travel without the support of the family is rarely physically, financially or culturally desirable.

The overall effect is that birth attendants are working in isolation, without opportunity to share experience or knowledge. A doctor will have little understanding of the traditional practices of the rural *dai* and the conditions under which she must work; similarly the *dai* knows little of the trained hospital-based staff in the cities.

The place of work

Although about 98 per cent of births take place in the home, alternatives are provided by the government, non-government organisations (NGOs) and the private clinics. The government provides the twelve district (teaching) hospitals, the Upazila Health Complexes (UHC) in the semi-rural areas, the maternal and child welfare centres (MCWC) and the family welfare clinics (FWCs) in the villages, from which outreach services are based. It is in these hospitals and clinics, where a mere 2 per cent of deliveries occur, that the trained staff are based. Attempts are being made to extend the services into the rural communities, but physical and cultural obstacles make this a time-consuming process.

Parallel to the hierarchy of birth attendants is their placement in the relative institutions. The maternity wards of the hospitals are staffed by male and female doctors, nurse-midwives, and occasionally FWVs. Basic nursing duties, such as bed-baths and bed pans, are not carried out by these members of staff, but by the relatives or *ayahs* that stay with the patient.

The extent to which the staff can practise, as in all medical institutions, is limited by both the training they have received and the facilities available. In Bangladesh the hospitals are faced with an inappropriate and outdated medical training. In addition maternal health, low on the government's list of priorities in an impoverished health system, receives negligible input. Basic supplies and equipment are provided mainly by the aid agencies. The staff, facing almost impossible odds, are highly skilled improvisers. Morale is low, however.

Disturbing scenes in the maternity wards of many of the hospitals are commonplace. The wards are overcrowded, hot and insanitary; women may have to share beds or sleep on the floor, wearing soiled saris often unchanged since before delivery, their babies wrapped in dirty rags. Women may be examined, or deliver, publicly. Attention to 'luxuries' such as screens or sterile equipment, let alone niceties such as routine postnatal care or health education, are unlikely where essentials such as water, electricity or working latrines are lacking.

Some maternity wards are able to provide special attention to the high percentage of women suffering from eclampsia or puerperal sepsis. Conditions are rarely ideal, as in one hospital in the four-bedded area for high-risk women, where six patients were lying, each having delivered. One woman, unattended, was having an eclamptic fit. She had delivered twins, one of which had died, the other of which was being held by a distraught student nurse who was administering unmonitored amounts of oxygen to the baby. The only doctor covering the ward was in theatre. The hospital had neither paediatrician nor paediatric equipment. The attendant relative responsible for purchasing drugs and supplies had gone for an untimely rest. Essentials such as suction, water or emergency drugs were not available.

When hopes for providing better services are frequently dashed by lack of facilities and staff, it is hardly surprising that birth attendants become too disillusioned to maintain such resuscitative attempts. It is indeed a tribute to the hospital-based birth attendants that they continue to provide as humane a service as possible under such stressful and demoralising circumstances.

The Upazila Health Complexes, large, purpose-built structures in semi-rural areas, are staffed as the district hospitals, but with fewer personnel. They have a general function in dealing largely with casualties, but a few beds are kept on the female general ward for maternity cases. Most women who go to them go for family planning, and they have unfortunately become disreputable centres for female sterilisations. Few normal deliveries take place in the UHCs, but they do have a function as referral centres for emergency obstetric cases. The main problems faced by them are that medical staff would, understandably, prefer to work in cities where potential for gaining greater experience and for promotion exists. Although administratively required, it is not really acceptable for women doctors to reside at the UHCs unless family are present, an unlikely situation. Supplies and equipment are minimal, and as a result services provided are basic. Emergency caesarean sections may be done under local anaesthetic. Fortunate patients, with relatives able to purchase intravenous fluids, may survive a haemorrhage, but without a blood transfusion. Survival of the fittest is the rule for the woman with eclampsia. The doctors who handle such cases are unlikely to have had previous experience with obstetric complications, and few are trained in the use of, for example, forceps. The role of the unsupported nurse-midwife, or family welfare visitor, is reduced to administering drugs, completing charts and the admission–discharge book.

The Maternal and Child Welfare Centres (MCWCs) are innovative in that they are staffed by women only, the family welfare visitors and trained traditional birth attendants. Sometimes a woman doctor is available. They are small, ten-bedded buildings with a 'clinic' room used for family planning or normal deliveries. The emphasis is on family planning, but they are friendly, and women who attend the antenatal clinics are encouraged to come for delivery. Any of the staff attend the delivery, but the FWV is responsible for identification of problems and subsequent referral to a UHC or district hospital.

The advantages of referral are, however, questionable. Not

only must availability of, and payment for, transport be taken into account, but consideration must be given to whether or not the site of referral can achieve anything that the MCWC (or FWC) cannot. A typical example is that of the case of a baby boy, born in an Maternal and Child Welfare Centre, the delivery having been conducted by a TBA. The baby was severely asphyxiated, and the FWV proved her resourcefulness by resuscitating the baby by mouth-to-mouth and a steroid injection, a wise move in the absence of suction, oxygen, or even water. It was clear that intensive paediatric care was required, and she carefully explained to the relatives that the baby should be referred to the district hospital, only ten minutes' walk away, where one of the few paediatric intensive care units was being established. The relatives were worried by the prohibitive costs of medication, thought they would be ignored in the hospital, and had little faith in what would be done. Eventually, they were persuaded to go. About twenty minutes later they returned, with the baby. Admission had been refused on the grounds that its condition was not serious enough to take up one of the few cots, and that limited equipment meant that there was little that could be done.

Given that this delivery occurred under supervision, in a clinic, and near a referral centre, it is understandable that attempts to transfer women and newborns with complications – during the monsoon floods or the heat of the drought, by rickshaw or boat – are rarely made.

The family welfare centres (FWCs) are small, rurally situated clinics. This is where the family welfare visitor (FWV) is based, along with other members of the 'primary health care' team, including a medical assistant (usually a man, with general medical duties) and a pharmacist. The FWV is herself provided with two basic kits, the family planning and the delivery kit. The responsibility for management and supplies is given to the well-named family planning officer (FPO), of purely administrative background. The efficiency of each FWC rests largely on the FPO, and a balance between his conscience and other temptations.

The daily business consists mainly of family planning routines: the insertion of Copper-T IUDs, the distribution of pills or condoms, and the performing of menstrual regulation. Sterilisation is done in some clinics where additional members of the sterilisation team are present. Antenatal care is provided by the FWVs with greater experience, as many are sadly lacking in basic skills such as palpating, taking blood pressures, or doing blood or urine tests. (Even more alarming is that few members of the clinic know how to use an autoclave, of which parts are frequently missing, or perform an aseptic technique.) In reality women are not encouraged to deliver there. Ideally the FWV should coordinate her work with the selected TBAs of that area. It is in the role of the trainer of the TBAs that the FWV is crucial, if progress is to be made. The more experienced and competent FWVs tend to have a better working relationship with the local TBAs, or *dais*, than do the young, poorly trained ones unfamiliar to the area, and with less experience of delivery than the *dais* themselves.

Other responsibilities of the FWV, such as satellite clinics, home visits, and even home deliveries, are not always physically possible. Payment for her safe transport is often not readily available. The FWV is caught between what the health planners would like to think she is doing and what the comunity, and her resources, allow her to do. The potentially ideal, trained, and rurally situated birth attendant is thus made virtually redundant in her contribution to safe delivery.

The NGOs, or non-government organisations, have greater access to and control of funds, and provide the best facilities for safe delivery. Through these organisations, such as the Save The Children Fund (UK), CARE (USA), and Rangpur and Dinajpur Relief Services, it has been proved that well-planned and practically thought-out basic training programmes, cheap, simple and appropriate locally produced TBA kits, in combination with national programmes, in particular the tetanus toxoid campaign, can drastically reduce maternal and infant mortality rates. The NGOs are also funding locally organised groups, such as the Bangladesh Women's Health Coalition and the Bangladesh Rural Advancement Committee, which are most effective in encouraging active participation of the local community. In addition attempts are being made to liaise with the government's national programme, rather than working in splendid isolation.

Private clinics are scattered throughout the major towns and are the choice of those who can afford to pay, as home delivery, even for the rich, has not been popular since the British medical influence. The clinics offer more privacy, better standards of hygiene, access to more facilities, and doctors who have usually trained abroad. 'Midwifery' staff are selected, and trained, by the doctors. Reputations vary, and it has been known for maternal and infant deaths to occur from lack of basic attention to asepsis, or tetanus toxoid administration. Private clinics do, however, have the potential, and responsibility, for raising the standards in the country.

Training potential for the birth attendants

The greatest hope for the future of birth attendants in Bangladesh is in the provision of good training. Birth attendants are, through personal experience, acutely aware of their need for more knowledge. The speed, and energy, with which for example FWVs and TBAs absorb information is a refreshing contrast to the attitude of the encumbered administration behind the training programmes. Doctors and nurse-midwives are similarly reaching out for more appropriate information.

The doctors unfortunately remain burdened with outdated British theoretical training and are without access to new books, literature or appropriate resources. The emphasis continues to be on medical management of hospital deliveries. 'Patients' are required to have routine procedures of that era (enemas, shaves and episiotomy) and to lie supine during labour and at delivery. Premature infants are separated from the mothers and fed bottled milk, and no effort is made to maintain lactation in the mother.

Medical students compete with nurse-midwives to gain the five or ten minimum deliveries they must conduct. It is possible for doctors to specialise in obstetrics and gynaecology, but it is not a popular choice, lacking not just the glamour but also the minimum facilities required to make it a satisfying job. For example Bangladesh does not yet have access to sonicaids, mechanical intravenous infusion counters for oxytoxic drugs, or epidurals, let alone sterile equipment or oxygen and suction in the rural clinics. The majority of doctors gain their experience in emergency deliveries of women who arrive in hospital in a critical condition. There is little time for students to work in the outpatient departments where antenatal care may be given, or to be trained in postnatal care and follow-up.

Attempts are being made through UNICEF-supported government programmes to revitalise a previous training programme, the aim being to train doctors to cope with the complicated cases referred to them at the semi-rural UHCs. Hopefully the medical school curriculum will, one day, be updated too.

The nurse-midwives face a similar dilemma in the legacy of their archaic training. Although the three-year nursing course is presently being upgraded with assistance from the World Health Organisation, the one-year midwifery training is without support. The nurse-midwives' role as active practitioners is negligible. In essence their jobs include ward management (no mean feat in overcrowded wards), recording observations and administering routine antibiotics. Tutors are rarely able to supervise training at ward level. Student nurse-midwives do not usually work in the antenatal clinics, nor do they gain any community training experience.

The training of the FWV, the woman with the enormous responsibility of training the TBAs in the villages, has received a relatively large amount of attention. The curriculum has been upgraded on several occasions, with the support of various agencies. She must, however, absorb an enormous amount of information in eighteen months, from basic principles of care to information on family planning, diarrhoea, infectious diseases, immunisations, care of the under-5-year-old, and so on. Approximately four weeks is allocated to safe delivery, and this takes the form of classroom-based lectures. Although many FWVs have an interest in childbirth, it is understandable that many are reluctant to take on so great a responsibility at village level.

The lack of time allocated to an issue of such national importance seems to reflect the lack of appreciation, by the government and the local aid agency health planners, as to what safe delivery, or being a birth attendant, is all about. Speed in implementation of programmes is, however, of the essence, and it has been felt that some effort, no matter how basic, is better than nothing at all. Attempts to compensate for the lack of skills training, in particular regarding delivery, are being introduced by making the 'refresher courses' practically based and by using a 'module' method for teaching the senior FWV, a new supervisory cadre. The 'module' method has been received with great enthusiasm by trainers and trainees. Of the ten weeks of the course, five are spent gaining practical experience in the Maternal and Child Health Training Institute, and the remaining five in selected village FWCs where practice is gained in, for example, how to teach TBAs most effectively. The trainees keep the modules as reference material. It is clear from the fervent interest shown by these trainees that they have, so far, been underutilised in their role as facilitators of safe delivery.

The national TBA training programme is a bold attempt by the government, with UNICEF support, to train one TBA for every village. There is no doubt that a successful programme will have an enormous impact in reducing maternal and infant mortality rates, and will go a long way to raise the socioeconomic status of the village women.

A new TBA training programme is at present being initiated alongside senior FWV, and FWV refresher training. Unfortunately the previous programme came to an abrupt halt when it became clear that administrative problems were making progress impossible. A positive outcome, however, was that a review of the 'failed' programme written by a midwife has highlighted technical problems faced by many such programmes in Third World countries, not only in Bangladesh. Recommendations included that more care should be given to the selection of the TBAs for training, that selection be done by the FWV (not the FPO and medical officers), that official criteria be established (i.e. age and number of deliveries done), and that two to three TBAs be trained for each village.

As far as the curriculum was concerned, it was suggested that consideration should be given to the TBA in her traditional role as a birth attender, and not as a healer, as well as to the fact that these women are illiterate and unused to formal teaching sessions. It was therefore recommended that the curriculum should be even more basic, concentrating only on safe delivery, care of the newborn, and breastfeeding. The training should be nationally standardised, and should use methods of demonstration and repetition; the flip-chart pictures should be clear and simple. Extra subjects, such as family planning and oral rehydration therapy for diarrhoea, should only be introduced at later follow-up sessions. The delivery kit should be more basic.

Previously TBAs had been so overwhelmed with information that they had been unable to grasp simple procedures such as handwashing and boiling the blade and cord tie. The extent of deviation from basics is apparent to the doctors when they are called to do emergency Caesarean sections on referred cases where TBAs have administered repeated intramuscular injections of oxytoxic drugs, causing ruptured uteruses and, often, stillbirths.

Encouragingly, the lack of support to and increasing workload of other birth attendants, namely FWVs and women doctors, were recognised. For the first time the inclusion of midwives in the programme was mentioned, as was lengthening training courses and making them more practically orientated.

Many of these recommendations have been taken into account in the new training programme. Work is still being done on standardising the curriculum with the cooperation of the numerous NGOs involved, and on focusing on safe delivery only. Progress is being made. The true potential for all levels of birth attendants is clearly visualised at the Azimpur Maternal and Child Health Institute in Dhaka. This hospital, although subject to the same limitations as all others, has proven that women themselves can provide the best care. The hospital is unique in that it is run by an all-women staff, it provides integrated family planning and maternal health services, emphasis is on preventative care though curative services are given, and training at all levels is available. This hospital has the largest number of deliveries per year, approximately 3,500, reflecting the confidence of the large catchment area.

It remains for the government and NGOs involved to take the opportunity now to provide coordinated and appropriate training programmes at all levels for birth attendants. The women are ready and waiting.

THE INFLUENCE OF INTERNATIONAL AID ON THE ROLE OF THE BIRTH ATTENDANT

One of the poorest countries in the world, Bangladesh is supported by massive injections of international aid money, which in the 1980s funded about 94 per cent of the country's public investment programme. As a result donor agencies have an extraordinary and unprecedented amount of control. Child-birth is no exception. The dire present-day situation is not just a reflection of the low socioeconomic status of Bangladeshi women, but of divisions and conflicts between major aid agencies, and resulting confusion over direction in the government.

The identification of the need for maternal health care has been emphasised by agencies such as UNICEF, the World Health Organisation, the British Overseas Development Administration (ODA), and the Save The Children Fund (UK); a large amount of funding also comes from Swedish, Dutch and Norwegian governments. With the support of UNICEF the government has chosen 'safe delivery', along with immuni-zation, control of diarrhoeal diseases, and family planning, as one of the four national priority programmes. Efforts are also being made to increase awareness that poor maternal health is linked to low socioeconomic status, as well as to factors such as illiteracy and nutritional habits. Much of this work is being done by local groups such as 'Nijera Kori' ('Do it Yourself') and 'Women for Women', involved amongst other projects in consciousness-raising. Such groups are also producing cheaper and more appropriate equipment, for example delivery kits for their TBAs.

The greatest setback to progress in maternal and child health has been the division between maternal and child health and family planning. The devastating political conflict between the aid agencies was caused by the artificial division of the two issues, making it administratively impossible to integrate maternal health with family planning. It resulted from the introduction, in 1983, of financial incentives to family planning workers. This decision was endorsed, and financed, by USAID (United States Agency for International Development) and the World Bank, and subsequently administered by the govern-ment of Bangladesh. The issue of incentives in a country of extreme poverty immediately raises moral and ethical questions regarding 'population control' as opposed to freely chosen family planning.

The direct effect of incentives is that the field workers,

influenced by the bureaucratic split in the hierarchy of control, have become divided in their priorities and unable to coordinate their work to reach the common goal. The reality is that field workers, including the FWV (and the client), are paid for family planning but not for other work such as maternal health or delivery. The FWV, the only member of the team who provides both, is in a pivotal position. The FWV receives not only more financial rewards for concentrating on family planning, but also more essentials like support, supplies, and equipment from the FPO than she would if she were to spend the recommended time on antenatal, delivery and postnatal cases, or on training TBAs. Staff are also penalised for not reaching family planning targets.

The system of incentives is now so deeply ingrained that it is difficult to imagine how other programmes will succeed without the use of financial rewards. The confusion within the government is understandable; as one official commented, 'It's not the donor's responsibility to supervise the government programmes. If you buy a car from me and then run someone over, is it my fault?'

The introduction of inappropriate technology, including inappropriate training courses, as well as the dumping of sophisticated, unusable and irreparable medical equipment that no one has been trained to use or maintain, has cost a great deal of time and money. As proved in the reviews of the TBA programme, and other training programmes, teaching TBAs to wash their hands is cheap and effective. Stockpiling of useless materials is more common, wasteful, and of benefit only to the donor nation. Examples are manifold, and include Bangladesh's only paediatric ventilator. Nobody knows how to use it, there is no blood gas machine to accompany it, and neither technician nor spare parts exist to maintain it. One district hospital has three operating theatres, two of which are idle, but in which is stored millions of dollars' worth of the latest equipment for refined obstetric and gynaecological surgery. Even if the expertise and the maintenance were provided, such facilities only benefit a tiny minority.

Research into what is being practised by birth attendants at village level, and into what facilities really exist, or are needed, is sorely lacking. Most of the data at present refer to family planning, and are collated by individual aid agencies. Such information is not always reliable; as one western adviser stated with reference to sterilisation, 'If people die during an operation, or there is a complication, their record cards will be torn up.' Maintaining records on births and deaths is a problem, and there is no national system for recording the number, type or outcome of deliveries. Some hospitals are without records altogether. Similarly, there does not yet exist a register of supplies, equipment or technical assistance available or required.

An adequate referral system is yet to be established, in particular to cope with the high rates of eclampsia, infection, haemorrhage and paediatric complications. Until this is done, training TBAs to 'refer such cases to the nearest health centre' is of little value. The number of administrators involved in the MCH/FP programmes seems vast, relative to the number of trainers, field workers and midwives who are actually providing the service. It appears that the aid agencies and the government have further compounded the legacy of British bureaucracy.

What can be done by the aid agencies?

In attempts to compensate for the demoralising effect of previous conflicts, and in the light of new information regarding TBA training, as well as the developing trend to support 'women's development' programmes, the more progressive aid agencies are working towards major improvements in the maternal health programme. These include expanding support by means of community education to women, strengthening the referral system, upgrading training facilities and curricula, and developing monitoring systems to measure the impact of these interventions.

In addition, aid agencies must take the responsibility for coordinating their efforts to provide a cohesive national programme based on shared experiences and knowledge. More research into the sociology of childbirth is required, and systems for recording information must be put into use before the existing situation is fully understood and effective planning can be achieved. Clarity as to what is the professional role of all birth attendants is required. Training must be appropriate and the position of the nurse-midwives must be raised so that, once they are recognised as practitioners in their own right, they can give support to others.

Last but not least, the involvement of 'midwives' and all birth attendants themselves is essential if any of the above far-reaching proposals are to be achieved. To date most of the responsibility has been taken by anyone from administrators to epidemiologists, but midwives have been noticeable only by their absence. Midwifery is little understood, and is not recognised as a profession by many members of the aid agencies, especially amongst those based in North America where the nurse-midwives are yet to regain their independent status. Sadly, it is common for midwives to have to renounce their profession for the more acceptable and competitive qualification of, for example, public health nurse, nutritionist, or statistician.

Bangladesh needs midwives now. Aid agencies must recognise that midwives are skilled professionals, and must use them as such to effectively promote the MCH programme as well as the status of all birth attendants in Bangladesh.

THE FUTURE CHALLENGE OF BIRTH ATTENDANTS

The challenge before the childbearing woman and the birth attendant has never been so great. Women of Bangladesh are experiencing a crucial time of change. 'Safe delivery' is, at last, a priority, and 'women's development' is being promoted.

Now that their welfare is being taken seriously, childbearing women must come together in self-respect and request help from the birth attendants. The birth attendants can now speak out, unite politically, share experiences, demand better training, and stand up for the fundamental rights of a women to a safe delivery. For what is more appealing to women, as childbearers or birth attendants, than to realise that they themselves, united, have the power to remove the threat of death from each childbearing woman and from one in five of their precious resource – children?

REFERENCES

T. Blanchet, *Women, Pollution, and Marginality in Rural Bangladesh*, Dhaka University Press, 1984.

J. Greenburg, *A Review of the National TBA Training Programme*, UNICEF, Bangladesh, 1984.

F.E. McConville, *An Assessment of Maternity Hospitals for Use in the Clinical Teaching of Safe Delivery*, UNICEF, Bangladesh, 1987.

Betsy Hartman and Hilary Standing, *Food, Saris and Sterilization*, Bangladesh International Action Group (BIAG), London, 1985.

MIDWIFERY AND RURAL HEALTH CARE IN GUATEMALA

AMANDA HOPKINSON

Guatemala is a country of approximately 109,000 square kilometres, the largest in Central America. Like Costa Rica, Panama and Nicaragua, it straddles both the Pacific and the Atlantic coasts. Also like them and in common with the Caribbean Basin as a whole, its principle exports are the 'three Cs', cotton, coffee and cane, although meat and fish are increasingly significant products. But unlike its regional neighbours, Guatemala is also still rich in natural tropical jungle, particularly dense in the north-west plateaus, where the rain forest alternates with wide lakes and sultry volcanoes.

One reason for the continuing existence of virtually uncharted regions within the *altiplano* (highlands) is a low population density. Although numerically Guatemala's population is the highest of any country immediately south of Mexico, the 8 million inhabitants are spread in a density of barely two per square kilometre, compared with El Salvador's 200. Between 5 and 6 million people are *indigenos*, native Indians of predominantly Mayan extraction although speaking at least twenty-three distinct languages, and each group has its own traditions, customs and dress. The entire *ladino* (white/hispanic) population is concentrated in the cities, particularly the capital, and the Indians' remoteness and the lack of land pressure have saved them historically from the fate suffered by so many of their relatives in neighbouring countries of being persecuted or hunted to extinction.

There is now a resurgence of anthropological and sociological interest in these indigenous traditions. As long ago as 1923, the noted Guatemalan author Miguel Angel Asturias observed the blurred divisions between native cultural, religious and medical/magical practices.[1] A great number of them he simply categorised as 'cults', those surrounding fertility being a particularly obvious example of mixing worship and witchcraft with primitive hygiene and medicaments. And as recently as September 1987, an indigenous Indian spokeswoman at the United Nations[2] complained, 'The government treats us like zoo animals, always sending in anthropologists and sociologists to observe our practices.'

The Indians' profound suspicion of what the *ladinos* send extends even to international family planning organisations such as APROFAM, financed by the International Planned Parenthood Federation of the United States. The borderline between the First World's exporting of progressive concepts of fertility control and childbirth, and its experimentation with dangerous products or clandestine sterilisation programmes, has frequently been a fine one. When it was found, during the military's infamous 'beans or bullets' campaign in the early 1980s, that tinned milk distributed to rural women contained sterilisation agents, outside aid agencies were blamed for extending the army's already genocidal campaign against the native population.

Where government health policies and international agencies may fail, local self-help organisations can sometimes succeed. ACSECSA (the Association for Education and Training for Health) is primarily run for and by indigenous Indian women, who remain within their communities. Rather than have a nurse or midwife from the town, dressed in a western-style uniform with a hat and badge, appear as a visitor on behalf of either the national health department or the nearest APROFAM clinic, ACSECSA workers dress in the vividly coloured head-dresses and *huipiles* (embroidered blouses) of their villages, speak the local language and remain in every sense a part of the community. Spanish is taught to all ACSECSA workers, not only as a means of understanding western medical technology but also as a tool for defending traditional practices. But the emphasis remains on infusing culturally acceptable practices (such as herbalism and a wholistic approach) with a new vitality and validity.

ACSECSA's work, in being thus community-based, treats the person as a part of his or her *pueblo* (meaning both a people and a place). Midwifery is not therefore a practice that has to do simply with delivering babies, but part of a process of health care provided for young women within the context of their family life, and for the infant well into the age when he or she is weaned, usually at 2 or 3.

Ironically, the woman who founded the organisation in 1979 is herself a North American, married to a Nicaraguan. The principles Maria Zuniga adopted closely follow the 'decoding' and 'consciousness-raising' group teaching practices devised by the Brazilian educator Paulo Freire and applied in his home country, where by 1964 over 2 million people were involved in over 20,000 discussion groups. Freire's primary intention was to give the poor a voice, first of all to express needs and then to collectively work out possible solutions. As he reported twenty years after devising his teaching systems, 'The dependent society is by definition a silent society. Its voice is not an authentic voice, but merely an echo of the voice of the metropolis – in every way, the metropolis speaks, the dependent society listens.'[3]

The effect of this 'demystification' led to direct action on the part of the peasants, and so to changes in land tenure and ownerships, followed rapidly by a new and positive approach to education and health care. In the words of a peasant thus liberated and enabled by the experience to speak 'consciously':

'Before the agrarian reform, my friend, I didn't even think "Why?", because it wasn't possible. We lived under orders. We only had to carry out orders. We had nothing to say. Now it's all different. I was happy because I discovered I could make words speak. Before we were blind, now the veil has fallen from our eyes.'[4]

Unfortunately for the Indian population, Guatemala has known no such thing as a systematic policy of agrarian reform, and the question of their dispossession of and displacement from the land is as fundamental to their health and well-being as it is to their work and livelihood. It is well over thirty years since any attempt at land redistribution at the expense of a few vastly wealthy landowners was made. This was during the ill-fated regime of

President Jacobo Arbenz, who allowed 100,000 peasants access to minor land ownership for the first time. In 1954 he was overthrown in a CIA-orchestrated coup and from then until 1986 Guatemala was ruled by a series of military juntas more concerned with waging a 'dirty war' against peasants and Indians (renamed 'communists' and 'subversives') than with dealing with the problem of Latin America's most unequal pattern of landholding. Six months after the inauguration of President Vinicio Cerezo in March 1986 (the first civilian president since Arbenz), a Guatemalan priest, Fr. Andres Giron, addressed a rally of 5,000 in the small southern town of Nueva Concepcion before the nation's television cameras and demanded an end to the country's poverty. The one solution, he counselled, was agrarian reform.

It was the application of Freire's techniques within the dire situation of the peasants' increasing landlessness that caused Maria Zuniga so many problems. In her contribution to a book entitled *Helping Health Workers Learn*[5] she outlined the necessary integration of Freire's approach with the particular Guatemalan context, and recommended teachers to be good organisers as well as health experts. She gave the following advice:

- Ask questions that are truly open-ended without hinting at the 'appropriate' reply.
- For discussion starters use words, pictures, or objects that are familiar and will spark ideas.
- Try to avoid stating your own opinions as much as possible or when doing so make it clear they are yours.
- Be prepared for discussion to go in directions you didn't expect.
- Welcome criticism or disagreement.
- Keep your language simple (do not use jargon and clichés).

Simply following such basic and straightforward advice is, particularly in Latin America, seen to be a provocative and dangerous activity, as Freire himself discovered in Brazil: within two years a change of government put a stop to all his schemes, the military massacred whole communities of his pupils, and he received death threats by way of 'encouragement' to leave for exile abroad. According to Maria Zuniga, even under the repressive military regime of General Lucas Garcia,

I continued my work training village health workers and promoters, using conscientization. After a devastating earthquake, in which we also lost our home, the government got even more repressive. . . . The disappeared increased from scores to hundreds, then thousands. Religious workers were a prime target, as were labor leaders. . . . I knew many of those murdered. Once I saw fifteen bodies hanging from a tree. After the Sandinista victory [in Nicaragua, July 1979], peasants were killed in Guatemala at random. I stood up for campesino demands and began having lots of problems.[6]

Like Freire she received death threats, but clung to the informative and consciousness-raising aspect of ACSECSA's work. But in 1980 her husband and children were forced to leave the country, and in 1981 she followed them to the Atlantic coast of Nicaragua. If she, with the relatively protected status of a foreigner, experienced such persecution, what chance for native rural Guatemalans, many of whom had to watch helplessly at the massacre of whole villages?[7]

MILITARY GENOCIDE AND WAR BY ATTRITION

Even without Guatemala's exceptionally violent recent history, its record of maintaining life and health among the indigenous population has been appalling. From the cradle to the grave native Indians fare substantially worse than the *ladino* population, and overall Guatemalans face the worst health prospects of any country in Central America. In the country as a whole, there is only one doctor for every 10,000 people; 70 per cent of them practise in the capital, Guatemala City, where a bare 25 per cent of the population reside. Even then, these doctors are heavily concentrated in the affluent suburbs and are of little service to the growing drift of *campesinos* (rural population) to the city outskirts in search of work, who have often been deprived of their smallholdings by the army. Such internal exiles are termed the *desplazados* (displaced persons).

Eighty-five out of 1,000 infants die in their first year, compared to 12 per 1,000 in the UK. Over 80 per cent of the surviving under-5s are severely malnourished. In July 1986 a UNICEF report baldly concluded, 'Guatemala has the worst infant mortality rate in Central America. Every day 115 Guatemalan children under five – that's five children every hour – die from such diseases as diptheria, whooping cough, tetanus, measles or polio.' In the *altiplano*, it was noted, infant mortality was put at double the national figure, at 160 per 1,000, although the Health Minister himself in 1986 acknowledged that in some areas it stood as high as one in five.

Vaccines exist to render all such deaths unnecessary. But, according to a recent publication,[8] 46 per cent of the population (3.67 million people) have no access to any form of officially recognised health care and the Ministry of Public Health and Social Assistance (equivalent to the British DHSS) covers less than a quarter of the population. While nationally there is one doctor to every 10,000 inhabitants, in the *altiplano* there may be as few as one for every 85,000. One doctor to 25,000 patients is a 'good' ratio. There is a scant one hospital bed per 1,000 inhabitants, although the armed forces and their families count nearer seventeen per 1,000 at their disposal. In the UK the proportion is 6.43 per 1,000 population.

As regards hygienic facilities, only 54 per cent of homes had drinking water in 1985. In smaller villages (fewer than 2,000 inhabitants), 39 per cent of the people were obliged to draw water from rivers or lakes; there was no piped water at all. Overall, only 49 per cent of houses had access to any sort of latrine, and a known housing shortage of at least 650,000 units meant large numbers of families crowded into insanitary shacks or slums with dirt floors and little light of any kind.

Official government spending on 'defence and security' is twice as high as on health, but unofficially it is recognised as being considerably higher. Between 1980 and 1983 (the latest date for which statistics are available) the health budget was actually cut by 35 per cent. Rural health centres, even where they exist, are notoriously badly stocked and frequently closed for lack of medical personnel. The attitude of the existing workers sent out from the cities is often overtly hostile to the Indians' long-standing practices, and confusions frequently arise when patients seek to combine these with what they can afford of medicines imported from the USA. Since prescriptions rather than medicaments are usually handed out, *campesinos* would rather bypass the whole intimidating process and go straight to the local pharmacist, where there is one, for both the medical opinion and the treatment. Neither the rural health centres nor the local chemists are seen as having a significant contribution to make to the whole matter of childbirth. Only 16 per cent of registered births receive medical attention.

TRADITIONAL HEALERS AND THE IMPORTANCE OF LAND

The 70 per cent of Guatemala's population classified as 'indigenous' (61 per cent of whom live in rural areas) are of predominantly Mayan extraction. Despite the richness of their more than a hundred dialects and the astonishing variety of the women's traditional *cortes* (tight skirts) and *huipiles* (blouses), each with a woven motif signifying the wearer's village origins, there is a substantial similarity in the ways of life of widely geographically dispersed communities.

Since the *conquistadores* deprived the Maya of their great cities and fertile lands, the Indians have spent the major part of the past 500 years in retreat, always moving to increasingly inaccessible mountainous areas. Nonetheless, as with their distant North American native relatives, they retain an attitude to the world (and specifically to the land and the corn it can grow) that holds religious significance as well as posing a continual political problem. This has major implications for health, particularly within the context of widespread maternal-infantile malnutrition. This culturally imprinted view of the world has some of the following characteristics:

- an integration of humans and the wider natural world;
- a strong sense of 'roots', of belonging to a particular locality and none other (this is a particularly poignant problem for the million Guatemalan internal exiles);
- a belief in the importance of maize as a source of fertility, sun and life. The great Mayan text, the Popol Vuh, sees humans as originally formed from an ear of corn;
- the sense of life as an ongoing cyclical process, which can

include reincarnation as well as the sense of the turning seasons;

- a belief that individuals are primarily part of a community and that their individuality is subsumed in this identity;
- a belief that children are gifts from the Place in the Sky, or Sky World, to which they return if they die young, and that each child is a whole person from conception onwards.

The integrity of even the unborn infant, for whom the staged development from embryo to foetus to baby is seen as but a gradual process of physical formation, lies in its earliest endowment with a *nahual*. Like the *huaca* of the Inca Indian, this is an individual natural element – it may be a wind, a grass or an animal – which functions as the child's guardian angel. The child will be raised to show special respect to his or her protector, and to seek endowment with its strengths and qualities. Given the importance of community and environment that surrounds the child's birth, it is an event endowed with ceremony.

There are two main forms of assistance available to Guatemalan women in giving birth. One is provided by the *comadrona*, a local woman and often a long-standing friend of the family, who has probably received very rudimentary training or none at all. Typically, she will help with all kinds of 'women's problems', from massage to relieve period pains to the use of herbs as abortefacients. When serving as a midwife, however, she usually also assumes a longer-term responsibility for the child, a role that combines elements of a health visitor's and a godmother's in overseeing the child's welfare.

The second form of available help is afforded by a *partera empirica*, a government-trained district nurse specialising in midwifery. She is unlikely, however, to have had more general medical training than a simple course in first aid. How familiar she is with traditional techniques of childbirth depends on the organisation she works with.

In some areas a witch doctor (*chiman* amongst the Mayan Indians, *curandero* to Spanish speakers) is also called if the mother or infant appears to be at risk. His role is primarily to offer prayers and sacrifices. Mayan villages usually have a communal *temaxcal*, or steam bath, and women in labour may be taken there to bathe. Among the Quiché Indians, the witch doctor ministers to a woman having difficulties in delivery by cleaving apart a black chicken and letting the blood flow down her head and breasts. As soon as the infant is separated from the mother and draws a first breath, she or he is taken under the witch doctor's protection.

Many rites surround the severance of the umbilical cord and these involve invoking protection from the Evil Eye. Among a community of Cachikel Indians in the Petén as recently as 1986, I met a woman who kept a chicken feather stuck to her newborn's forehead as protection against the Evil Eye. A whole ceremony can attend its placing there, in which the witch doctor passes burning candles over the baby's head in the sign of the pagan cross while invoking long life and good health.

The traditional midwife attends to all kinds of 'women's complaints', delivers babies and performs abortions. (According to an early Spanish chronicler, Bernardino de Sahagun, the earth/fertility goddess she represented was 'worshipped by doctors and surgeons and bloodletters and midwives who also prescribed herbs to procure abortions').[9] To indicate the continuity of her role and the multiplicity of her tasks, let us take a contemporary example from neighbouring El Salvador:

> When the woman of the family gets sick . . . it is the *tortillera* who supplies the daily bread. The village *tortillera* makes the bread of God. She is also the official suppliant, the masseuse, anaesthetist, remover of worms from babies' stomachs, birth attendant, teacher of the Christian faith, and the one who teaches children how to read and write. She knows the mystery of herbs for curing sickness.[10]

Many of the midwife's roles and rites are common not only throughout Central America but in the Caribbean islands as well. In the Todos Santos highlands the midwife hangs the umbilical cord outside the child's home for twenty days, and mother and baby are ritually bathed in the *temaxcal* daily. When the period is up, the cord, some hairs from the infant's head and some geranium flowers are borne in procession to a site of pre-Colombian ruins blessed by the witch doctor. He prays over the burial of the relics, which are then covered with a stone which should thereafter remain untouched by others; otherwise bad luck will befall the child.

More commonly, and in many countries, the cord is buried beneath a tree or a plant that then becomes the child's own adoptive 'home'. Should the child grow up to travel, she or he needs to discover as similar as possible a new tree and sit beneath it to commune with the one at home. As soon as she returns home, respects must be paid to the original tree. And according to Ixquic, an indigenous women's organisation whose publications speak of native customs,

'When a boy or girl child is born, we bury the umbilical cord in the earth, and we go to the stream and say to it "Here is a new life which will need your water", we go to the volcano and say to it "Here is a new being that needs your protection", we go to the trees and say to them "Here is a new being that needs your shade" . . . and so we go to all of Nature saying "We present our children to you".' (from the testimony of María, a native Indian woman).

The principle is much the same as that of the *nahual* (guardian spirit). In return for paying respects to the tree, the child seeks some of its qualities – beauty, fruitfulness, strength. The tree's name may also figure among those of the child and the whole naming ceremony is in itself of symbolic significance, for the name is inextricably linked to the soul; if a child dies nameless, the soul perishes and cannot join its forefathers. With the integration of Roman Catholic practices, local patron saints are added to the list of ancestors and community names and, when a child has grown up in the north-west of the country, the child's birth date taken from the Tzolkin Calendar is also added.

The rituals surrounding the cutting of the umbilical cord may mask a very real danger, however. Where no midwife or community nurse is present with a properly sterilised 'gillette', women have to resort to potentially infectious instruments. In some parts of the country it is customary for a woman to go into the countryside and give birth by herself; she will cut her own cord with whatever is available – a shard of glass or pottery.

A frequent consequence of using unsterile implements is the

baby's infection with tetanus. According to a recent report, 'death due to tetanus represents between 23% and 72% of all neonatal deaths', and while 'infection of the umbilical stump is not always obvious varying from a minor infection to a gross sepsis . . . the case fatality rate in the neonatal group is as high as 85%.'[11]

One further curious dimension to the relatively high incidence of this entirely preventable (but so often fatal) disease among Indian babies is the increasing evidence that tetanus only arrived with the *conquistadores*; it did not exist in indigenous communities before the arrival of the Spaniards. Then it became known as the 'seventh day disease', for it habitually strikes infants when they are between three and twenty-one days old; a Dutch physician noted the Indians' use of copaíba oil to sterilise the end of the cord in an attempt to avert it. Reports also exist from the seventeenth century of cotton flowers being used with camphor to prevent 'the horrible mal', but by the eighteenth century churchmen were weighing in with their own theories. One held that such neonatal deaths could only be due to a delay in baptism; another to the force of original sin.

Just as change in birth customs which introduced the disease may have been brought by the *conquistadores*, so Spain had to provide possible solutions. Following mass neonatal deaths in 1795, the Royal Order in Aranjuez reported that 'a method of prevention for the "seventh day disease" has been found'. On its recommendation the king ordered the use of 'stick oil' (balsam of the copaiba/camibar tree) applied to the umbilicus. And in 1813 the church's recommendation was 'to baptise in warm water at any season' to avoid the ten-day risk period.

Further rituals attach to water after birth. Apart from a minimal cleaning up, the mother is expected to abstain from washing for forty days after her delivery. She also avoids sexual relations for that period. Similar superstitions have applied until recently throughout Europe and North America, and medical advisors still recommend abstaining from sexual intercourse until after a postpartum examination (usually six weeks after delivery). After forty days, a woman may take a steam bath or heat water on a brazier, and another member of her family, usually a woman or one of the children, will massage her back with seeds from the *alucema* or *cubanis* plant, which release a soothing oil. From this comes the rural saying, which I have heard repeated many times, 'For an instant of pleasure, nine months of travail, forty days of abstinence and five years of rocking the cradle.'

Five to seven years is the length of a childhood. The baby's principle nourishment for several years will be the mother's milk. Drinks made from maize or cocoa are believed to increase the mother's lactation, and steps are taken in the higher mountainous regions to ensure that her milk doesn't 'turn sour' or 'get cold'. In the border province of Huehuetenango, for example, women heat rocks and place them within hollowed boulders to warm their homes before nursing the child. A warm atmosphere helps the milk to flow freely.

Once past the age of about 6, children are integrated into the household as workers, boys always being considerably more prized than girls. In the countryside, where the average number of children to a family is seven or eight, parents who have only girls (or 'gourds' as they are sometimes scornfully called) are pitied or despised, while a father of many sons is regarded as a 'real man'. Many sayings assert the primacy of masculinity, from the father's role ('a woman bears the number of children her man decides') to the son's ('a son is born with his daily bread beneath his arm'). As one local woman wrily pointed out, 'If that were true, I'd be owner of a whole bakery by now.'

According to Indiana Torres, a doctor who has worked in maternal-infant child care in a number of state-run hospitals serving the poorest regions,

'While it is true that we saw a self-selecting tiny percentage of births – in many areas over 90 per cent may be entirely unattended – it is still possible to generalise about the indigenous women's attitudes. In the main, it is stoical. Often young girls are abandoned by their lovers if they become pregnant – almost invariably if the man is in the army. Marriage is much less significant, and even lifelong couples may well be unmarried, and even if they are men take the attitude that pregnancy and birth are a woman's business. The women hide their pregnancy under a shawl (*faja*) and work until the last minute, drop the baby and return to work almost at once. They squat for the delivery, almost never cry out, and expect little by way of assistance. If a village *comadrona* (midwife) attends, it is primarily her presence that is of help and support. She may offer the woman a pimiento infusion to stimulate contractions and the later expulsion of the placenta, or massage the mother's abdomen with castor oil to help press the baby's head against the cervix and ease crowning. But she may primarily be there to give moral support, saying prayers and passing lit candles over the mother's body.'

Olga Escobar, who also works with rural women and their children, points out that both a traditional *comadrona* and a trained *partera empirica* may employ pre-Colombian and early Hispanic rites for the child's well-being, for example in the repeated passing of a hen's egg over the newborn's body to 'absorb evil humours', or the placing of wads of tobacco under the child's *petaque* (sleeping mat) to cure fevers. Once used, both the egg and the tobacco will be re-instructed to relieve the child of the ailment and then thrown away over the *comadrona's* left shoulder. Sometimes, however, symptoms are recognised that we also know are dangerous. If a baby's fontanelle begins to sag, for example, women of the Chimaltenango and Quetzaltenango regions tip the child upside down and bang the soles of her feet. It would help more if they rapidly attempted to get the baby to drink and retain more fluids, as a depressed fontanelle is a sign of dehydration.

According to Olga, most ailments are thought to come from the Evil Eye. Not satisfied with introducing a variety of illnesses and humours, the Eye keeps a particular watch on good-looking babies who have to be protected at all times. They are given tiny coral bracelets or, later, rubber or liquorice root to chew. The Evil Eye can also be turned upon a newborn by the presence of a drunken man or a menstruating woman, both of whom are expected to keep their distance.

Pregnancy is also regarded as a potentially fraught time of life and pregnant women should not step upon anything that rests on the floor, including mats or bedding, but walk around or remove it. Otherwise the baby may be born with the cord around his or her neck. The woman should also refrain from beating eggs or grinding maize for porridge or her cooking will spoil. While such beliefs have much in common even with Talmudic laws, in Guatemala good humour – or ribaldry – attaches to spotting a woman whose cooking batter goes stringy instead of fluffy or whose pancakes turn out lumpy.

The moon is closely linked to menstruation and fertility. While it is dangerous to conceive during the first quarter it is worse for a pregnant woman to see the moon at this stage, or rather to be seen by it. She must stay indoors until the moon is waxed at least half full; otherwise a miscarriage can result. And should there be an eclipse, she must wear a pair of scissors, a knife or another piece of metal at her waist to avoid a birth defect.

With such an emphasis on the hazards of being observed, whether (in the woman's case) by the moon or (in her child's) by the Evil Eye, it is understandable that women resist being medically examined or 'seen' either pre- or postnatally. In Indiana Torres's experience,

'They are not only very stoical but very secretive. Children are not taught the facts of life, and their parents do not wish them to have sex education in schools. Women learn from other women how babies are born. We mave won a major battle in persuading *comadronas* and training *parteras empiricas* to always travel with their pots for boiling water, their scissors and cloths which they must sterilise. And many of the traditional teas and oils do help a mother in labour. But the prevalent beliefs, whether in the pagan Evil Eye or a more Christian "chastisement of God", generate a fatalism in the face of avoidable infant mortality. This combines with a hopelessly inadequate system of health care where even existing rural health centres may only be visited by a doctor once a week or a month, to prevent us making the headway we could.'

Indiana's point is that so long as the *parteras empiricas* receive only minimal training, doctors are essential to attend births where complications may arise.

HEALTH PROMOTERS AND ACSECSA*

It was in the context of 500 years of Spanish colonisation and a particularly brutal series of military dictatorships from the 1950s

* The Association for Education and Training for Health.

on that a whole 'health promotion' campaign was born. This grew up out of a complex structure of non-government organisations backed by charities, churches and international aid agencies. Many arrived in the wake of the devastating 1972 earthquake, sent in from abroad as emergency troubleshooters, who swiftly discovered that Guatemala's health problems were endemic as well as temporary, and in both cases involved avoidable epidemics that rendered the country 'the sickest in all Latin America'.

Because of the lack of any kind of an adequate infrastructure, new alternatives had to be tried to meet the needs of the poor. These involved combining preventative primary health care with traditional Mayan remedies based on treatment with herbs and massage, and a wholistic approach. The relief agencies – unlike the government – recognised that to make this function villagers needed to volunteer from within a local community, and to harness their traditional knowledge to simple diagnoses and treatments of major infections. The main causes of premature death are gastric infections, tuberculosis, whooping cough, malnutrition and perinatal mortality. Preventative health care here highlights the need for a combination of simple modern technology (such as vaccination programmes) and traditional customs and diet.

The importance of food is linked into a religious cycle around maize-growing ceremonies and the phases of the moon. Each stage of the corn's growth has its own name and its own god or goddess, from the seed to the fully sprouted ear. Just as the seasons are marked on a calendar based on the phases of sun and moon, so a pregnancy is counted through 'nine moon cycles', each one notched on the trunk of a tree, often the one to which the child will be dedicated and one where the ancestors may be buried.

Despite the many rites that surround the production, cooking and serving of corn-based meals, few Indians can now eat even the fruit or vegetables they may harvest themselves. The staple diet is of *tortillas* (unleavened bread made of maize and water), with the possible addition of red beans for protein and salt for flavour. All else has to be sold, for whereas the basic living wage for an average family is over $12, the minimum rural wage is barely $3, with many landowners paying well below. But the problem of growing even a small amount of additional products to market is continually exacerbated by an iniquitous land tenure system, whereby 4 per cent of the population own 60 per cent of the land, and a mere 2 per cent own 80 per cent of all cultivable land.

ACSECSA began establishing local groups in the mid-1970s, and was formally established in 1978, to start functioning the following year. It decided upon a three-pronged approach, offering therapies, education and administrative back-up through the opening of clinics, dispensaries and the setting up of *comites de promotores* (cooperatives of health promoters).

While part of the thrust of providing medical treatment came through direct deals with major drug manufacturers in order to provide low-cost, non-brand-name medicaments, the intention was also to incorporate knowledge of herbal remedies proper to each particular region. Within seven years ACSECSA had seventy-two groups operating over the entire country, was publishing its own handbooks and testing and evaluating the groups' own remedies.

Health promoters are trained for one week a month over a three-month period. During this training they too are expected to contribute from their own knowledge, bearing in mind that it was the Maya who first used quinine to reduce fevers, teas to soothe gastro-intestinal complaints and labour pains, and guayaco for syphilis (it became a significant European import in the 'poxy' eighteenth century). Classes combine this input with new information, and on the day I visited ACSECSA's mother project in Chimaltenango, Manuela Alvarado was taking a class on 'Our Culture and Traditions'. She explained her work:

'We have to clearly distinguish between what is our history and what is part of our living culture. We may no longer believe in sympathetic magic, but we know how if we are angry with someone we may build up a headache until we express that anger – and if we shout too loud we may leave *them* with that headache! No more do we believe in illness as the vengeance of the gods of maize or the climate, but we know how ill winds blow no good and the diseases we acquire from poor food.'[12]

One of the greatest problems is the lack of a traditional connection between cause and effect. Like the Chinese, the Maya tend to believe in a synchronicity of events. This means, for example, that parents must be helped to understand that their babies can become ill through poor hygiene or that a nursing mother may not be producing 'bad milk' but be suffering from an inadequate diet herself.

Simple diagrams indicate hygienic precautions and the disease chains with the use of cartoons (there is over 80 per cent illiteracy among Indian women). The emphasis is on incorporating the *curanderos* (witch doctors) and *parteras* as health promoters, or as one of ACSECSA's founders, Antonia Castro de Ortiz, puts it, 'as a human resource and not as a source of conflict'. This is where they feel many of the 'official' nurses, supplied both by the Health Ministry (in scarce numbers) and by the US-financed family planning organisation APROFAM, fail: 'They are obviously from outside and want only to teach and not to learn, and the doctors are notoriously more interested in their own salary than in our health. We speak as one *indigena* to another, as equals. We're a channel for the people to use.'

Since ACSECSA refused to work in the government's 'model villages' and 'poles of development'[13] and publishes its first aid manuals in Cachiquel and Quiché (the major Indian languages), it receives no Health Ministry funds. Manuela Alvarado continues,

'Although we receive a small amount of independent funding, our approach is in fact very low-cost. Although we run clinics and dispensaries, we often meet in private homes and win people's confidence in small ways. We also work with the whole person within the whole family: we care for the mother through the pregnancy, assist at the baby's birth, then monitor the child's development through nutrition programmes and preventative health care.'

Such practices can be dangerous, and in Guatemala the challenge of midwives, rural nurses and health promoters has a particular context. As Antonia, one of the ACSECSA workers, explained,

'We cannot discuss diet without reference to employment and to land. We only have to issue diagrams of how to construct a latrine and we're trespassing on the *ladino* stereotype of the "dirty Indian" who wants to stay that way. Yes, our women breastfeed until the infant is well past walking, but how can we explain the inadequacy of this when it results from the woman's own malnourishment?'

Let us return to Freire and the risks of raising even simple but basic questions relating to the all-prevailing social injustice. Even ACSECSA's symbol, although underscored with an 'Approved by the Government Ministries' stamp, can be construed as a provocation, showing as it does a peasant on a ploughed field, wielding a spade and a manual before the high mountains of the *altiplano*. While ACSECSA's newsletter gives publicity to the government's rare 'vaccination days' with graphic illustrations of children afflicted with polio or measles, other articles describe herbal remedies and their counter-indicators and give prominence to (foreign) doctors who state their case for them, with such information as, 'Once removed from nature, man gradually loses also his health. . . . Instead of offering "cures", prescribing "remedies" to stifle symptoms, we should return to a lifestyle directed towards a healthy digestion, normal breathing and a clear skin.'

This may have a commonplace, even antiquated, ring in the west. We are by now used to being exhorted to rediscover a herbalism, homeopathy or holism otherwise lost in our culture. But in Guatemala such traditions remain as a pervasive force, and are all too frequently treated as a subversive one. Since 1980 500 health promoters and over seventy medical professionals have been killed (or have 'disappeared') by the armed forces.[14] According to an interview conducted in 1985,

A health promoter . . . works not only in health programmes but becomes more a social promoter, a more holistic health promoter. . . . However many of them have been accused by government forces of collaborating with the guerrilla, of being subversives . . . and this means death, disappearance or exile.[15]

The type of work undertaken by ACSECSA and its fellow organisations is unique in Central America. But then so too are conditions within Guatemala, with its predominantly indigenous population and 'ethnocidal' military. Within this context local people in small communities are encouraging the establishment of herb gardens, revitalising the practice of baby massage and gradually restoring people's control over their lives and health. In a single count taken in June 1986, it was found that 106 rural health centres built between 1978 and 1982 had never been opened for lack of staff and resources. In the same month San Juan de Dios, the capital's largest hospital, refused further admissions on the grounds that it would be 'professionally irresponsible' to take more patients. For three months, the hospital had been in crisis, and was left with barely five days' medical supplies and only meagre rations of cotton wool, bandages and antiseptic. The Health Ministry refused to act.

The problem for the health promoters is that they are not supposed to act either. It is not possible to be 'simply' a midwife in a rural zone and ignore the surroundings that must influence the new child's whole future and potential. Or, in the words of the great Salvadorean doctor Roberto Castillo, 'In a country with such problems, a prescription for health would have to start with a new social system in order to have a new health system.' By challenging the sociopolitical structure through raising general questions of hygiene or malnutrition, health promoters, and community midwives among them, are contributing to more than just the birth of a new generation.

NOTES

1 Miguel Angel Asturias, *El Problema Social del Indio*, 1930; revised and reprinted in Paris, 1971.
2 Rigoberta Menchu, in an interview with the author, September 1987.
3 Quoted in J. Benseman 'Paulo Freire, A Revolutionary Alternative', *Delta*, vol. 23, November 1978, pp. 27–40.
4 Paulo Freire, *Pedagogy of the Oppressed*, London, 1972.
5 David Werner and Bill Bower (eds), *Helping Health Workers Learn*, Washington, 1976.
6 Quoted in Ron Ridenour *Yankee Sandinistas*, New York, 1987, p. 23.
7 See Victor Montejo, *Death of a Guatemalan Village* (Willimantic, Ct., 1987) for a first-hand account.
8 *'Bitter and Cruel . . .' Report of a Mission to Guatemala by the British Parliamentary Human Rights Group*, London, October 1984.

9   From Luis A. Seggiaro, *Medicina Indígena de América*, Buenos Aires, 1969, p. 28 (my translation).

10 Manlio Argueta, *Cuzcatlán*, London, 1987, p. 103.

11 WHO reports, cited in Indiana Torres's thesis on 'Neonatal tetanus in Latin America', School of Hygiene and Tropical Medicine, University of London, 1987, p. 5.

12 Interview, from which all subsequent ACSECSA quotations are also taken, conducted in March 1986.

13 'Poles of development' are zones of control where the military supervises forced relocation of the native villages and Spanish is the only language allowed. The *ladinos'* suspicion of the indigenous population is so great that these 'concentration camps', as they are known to the locals, are a means of breaking up the Guatemalan guerilla movement and with it the traditional social communities.

14 From *Guatemala Health Rights Support Project Report*, Washington, 1986.

15 Quoted in an article by Maire Kenny entitled 'Risking lives for health', *Central America Report*, Spring 1987.

INTRODUCTION

DENMARK

In Denmark midwives are central to the system of care in childbirth. The Danish woman attends a midwife clinic five times during her pregnancy, her GP's surgery three times, and the antenatal department of an obstetric unit twice.

Midwives have retained the tradition of family-centred birth, and a woman may choose to have her partner, other relations and children with her during labour and at the birth. She is able to decide for herself the delivery position which she finds most comfortable.

Denmark, along with Finland and Sweden, has one of the lowest perinatal mortality rates in the world. It also has one of the lowest induction rates, and low vaginal operative delivery and Caesarean section rates.[1]

NOTE

1 J.M.L. Phaff (ed.), *Perinatal Health Services in Europe* (World Health Organisation), Croom Helm, 1986.

MIDWIVES IN DENMARK

SUSANNE HOUD

15.5.87

It is Saturday morning. The phone rings and it is one of my clients calling: 'I think I am in labour, I have had contractions for two hours. I feel good, don't hurry.' An hour later, after a nice bike ride, I am in the house. She, her husband and her 5-year-old son greet me. We know one another from several antenatal visits at their home. Four hours later she gives birth on her hands and knees with her husband in front of her, her son almost under her and me behind her. When the baby is born we all lift it through her legs and place the girl in front of the three of them. Slowly the mother sits down and lifts the child up to her breast.

In the week that follows I visit them almost every day. And life goes on – the birth is far behind us all, the daily chores are filling up their time and my time. The birth was important, but a normal event in their lives and mine.

22.6.87

Today is my birthday. I am on duty at the hospital. After five years doing research, I am back 'on the floor'. I am assigned to birth room no. 2. This couple is having their first baby. Her sister is there, she has just had a baby herself. The woman is in labour. Half dilated. Between contractions I introduce myself and tell them that I will be looking after her until 4 p.m. The three of them are a unit, having spent the long night hours together. They hardly talk, it is not necessary. The wet cloth is there, ready when she needs it, and the husband and sister change places to rest a bit every now and then. The long night shows in their faces and for them time is non-existent. I feel almost like an intruder. They accept my presence as long as I am quiet, which I am. She has the baby at 2 p.m. It is a girl and they forget that they are exhausted.

Two hours after the birth I say goodbye to them, tell them it is my birthday and that it is a fine day to be born on. I never see this family again.

Over the last few years I have worked in both settings, sometimes in the same week, attending home births on a private basis. Every time I shift from one setting to the other, I cannot help asking myself the question, is one way better than the other? And, how do I feel working the one way or the other way?

It is difficult to say where I feel most at ease and what is best for the family. The main issue here is that the family feels secure, relaxed, trusted and respected. In order to do that, the midwives taking care of them must be extremely sensitive and find out who they really are, if they only meet one another in the birth situation. Sometimes it works and sometimes it does not. It is a very fragile system.

Personally, I have no doubts about the way I like to work. I prefer to know the people I am dealing with during pregnancy and birth. Working in this way is a constant evaluation, a constant learning process. When I work in the centre, where I rarely meet 'my own' people, I can find myself escaping from the birth room to the cosier atmosphere of coffee drinking and small talk with the other staff in the staff room. I feel more drained after eight hours in the centre than after sixteen hours with people I know. And I feel lonely and sometimes burned out to a degree that scares me. Of course there are the good births where you 'swing' with the couple right away. You have energy, they have their baby when you are there, and you manage to go and see the woman twice on the postpartum ward to 'talk the birth through'. And I dance home. It is both interesting and frustrating to know how the surroundings influence my experience as a midwife. I am not the same midwife when I am with unknown clients in the hospital as I am with clients in their homes. Suddenly my colleagues in the hospital become more important for me than the woman in labour. It is a very subtle process, but it still happens. I hear myself say things, or not say things, which afterwards surprise me. I am very much aware of how far I can go within the framework I work in. The rules are there, some are written down and some are not. They can be changed, though, if you take the trouble. But how did we come here and how did it all start?

WHERE DO MIDWIVES COME FROM?

The Danish word for midwife is 'earth-mother'. The word has arisen from the fact that, in the old days, the birth took place on the ground and the midwife lifted the child from the ground. The word mother is there, because the midwife needed to be a mother herself, with her own birth experiences. The reason why it was important to give birth on the ground was probably that it was thought that the child got strength from the life-giving earth.

We know little about midwives before the sixteenth century. We can only guess that many women were usually present at a birth, all having had children themselves so that the total knowledge was as great as possible. One of the women had to be the midwife. The basis for this choice is difficult to guess. The earliest description of the midwife's role was written in 1510 by a doctor. It is a document about how impossible and useless the midwives are. He particularly complains about the midwives' harshness towards the birthing women. Priests, too, were keeping an eye on the midwives and, after the reformation, were supposed to educate them. There was concern that the midwives would use witchcraft but there are no accounts of any midwife being burned as a witch. From 1683 the doctors were also supposed to educate the midwives. This is ironic, since doctors had little knowledge about births at that time. Although very few accounts of birthing were written down, one or two exist. The following is an account of a birth on a small Danish island, Aeroe, about 100 years ago.

When Synne knew she was pregnant, she started to prepare for the birth. The house had to be tidied up – everything had to be cleaned and it was necessary to bake, slaughter and brew more than usual. A birth was a great event and should be prepared for properly.

When Synne felt that the labour had started, she sent for the 'helping-women' and the midwife. The helping-women knew that the time had come and they were ready. It was an honour to arrive first and each woman hurried. When the helping-women arrived, they saw Synne walking up and down the floor in the room. Her husband had gone and now the room belonged to the women. Synne's helpers put the water on to boil, each took a chair and sat in a circle. When Synne had her first urge to push, she sat down on the lap of one of the women with her back to the helping-woman and her feet on a small stool. The helper folded her hands around Synne's big stomach and then Synne and the woman pushed together. When the contraction was over, the woman went out of the circle and took out food. Coffee was made and jugs of beer and wine were passed around. Synne went from lap to lap in the helpers' circle. When the midwife arrived, she washed her hands in hot water and examined Synne. When Synne gave birth, she was sitting on the lap of one of the women, while the midwife was sitting inside the circle on a small stool in front of Synne. The three women all sat down at the moment of birth. Then Synne was helped to bed with her newborn child and much later, when all the women had celebrated the child's birth, the husband was called in.

Over the last hundred years birth has changed from being a women's event to a family event, with the men taking an active part in the birth, both on professional and personal levels. The place of birth has shifted too, from home to hospital. During the 1960s women complained that they were not able to give birth in hospital if they expected a normal birth. Their complaints, together with a need to centralise places of births, meant that there was suddenly room for everybody in the hospital or in the clinics, and in a very few years most births in Denmark took place in hospital. By the end of the 1960s 50 per cent of children in some areas of Jutland were still born at home, but by the mid-1970s this was no longer the case. The next step was that smaller units, with fewer than 100 births each year, were closed down. Only a few of these units are still working. Until 1973 midwives worked as district midwives employed by the county, with around 100 births each year, or in private practice, sometimes with 200 or 300 births a year. The midwives usually worked alone, on call night and day, at New Year and Christmas too. Although the job is very rewarding, it is a tough life. As a third year midwifery student I worked 'on the district' for a month in Jutland, where nearly 50 per cent of births were home deliveries. My midwife was Mrs Hansen. She had been there for twenty-five years and was now helping the second generation into life. She was quite an impressive person and she referred to her husband as Mr Hansen. In the month I spent with her we attended fifteen births. Ten babies were born at home and five in hospital. The first ten days went by without any births at all. We spent the time working at the antenatal clinic and making postpartum housecalls. I began to think that this sort of life was rather comfortable. Then it happened. For three days we were working almost all the time, stopping only for one or two hours' sleep every now and then. When Mrs Hansen called me for the fourth birth in three days, I almost cried from tiredness, but there was no way I could rest. During these long hours with her I got my first real feeling of what midwifery is truly about: sensitivity, love, patience and silence. Most of all I remember the silence. Hours could pass without a word. Mrs Hansen always stayed right next to the woman having a child; sometimes she would snatch some sleep in the other half of the double bed. She radiated calmness and warmth, and women trusted and respected her. She taught me always to believe what a pregnant woman said: 'If she calls you, then go and see her, no matter how insignificant she makes it sound; remember she had to pull herself together to pick up the phone and she would not do that if it was not necessary.'

In 1973 Mrs Hansen's era was over. A new centralised system was introduced. All midwives were employed by the country's social and health system, who were responsible for the care of the normal pregnant and birthing women. The midwives were organised in groups of between three and forty, determined by the size of the hospital where most of the births would take place. Each centre had an administrative leader who was very often part-time administrator and part-time midwife. The bigger units had leading midwives who were more concerned with professional matters. In each county there was a county midwife who worked closely with the social and health group in the county on health planning. This is the way the midwives still work. It is important to note that they are working in both primary and secondary fields of health care. Unlike some countries where one group of midwives work in the antenatal clinic and another group in the labour wards, each Danish midwife will work once a week in her (or his) antenatal clinic and spend the rest of the week on duty in the hospital or on call for home births. I worked for a while at an average midwifery centre on two big islands in the south of Denmark, and set up 'my' antenatal clinic in a health house in a small town in the north of one of the islands.

There were four GPs, the health visitor and laboratory worker in the health house. I was there once a week doing antenatal checks in the morning and attending housecalls in the evening, either to pregnant women or to women and families who had had their babies. I also ran antenatal classes the same day at the local school with my own clients from the antenatal clinic. For the rest of the week I would be on call for births, whether at home or in hospital. I seldom attended 'my own women' giving birth, but when I did I always enjoyed it very much. In Copenhagen there are few antenatal clinics and those that do exist are usually connected to a hospital. The idea of this central organisation is clearly to separate the centre from the hospital clinic. If the midwife or the GP diagnosed a problem, they could recommend that the woman go into a hospital clinic. There are only large delivery wards in Copenhagen and the midwives rarely leave the hospitals. The health centre system is potentially very flexible but currently, due to a lack of resources, it is not used to its fullest. The system was built to make continuity of care possible, which at the moment only happens during pregnancy. There could be continuity of care during birth if more resources were allocated. Several midwives have come up with ideas of mini-centres which could be built into the centre system if more midwives were employed.

THE CONTENT OF MIDWIVES' WORK

When the system of central organisation was introduced in 1973, a set of guidelines was developed for care during pregnancy, birth and the period after birth. The guidelines placed women in groups according to the risks involved in their pregnancy and were devised to help GPs decide whether a woman was at any risk and therefore should be referred to hospital early. Once designated 'high-risk', a woman would find it hard to get rid of the label. It would be the deciding factor in the number of visits she had from the midwife, for example, and would remain on her notes for the rest of that pregnancy. After a few years it became obvious that there were 'low'-risk groups (such as women over a certain age) and 'high'-risk groups (women with diabetes for example). Midwives, parents and doctors started to question the risk system. In 1983 the Minister of the Interior, a woman, requested that the guidelines for perinatal care be revised. Revisions were suggested by the obstetricians but these focused only on the risks or dangers of pregnancy and birth, so she requested advice from the World Health Organisation. We, the midwives, could only agree with her. The next step was to send the obstetricians' suggestions to a wide range of people, including user organisations, midwives' and nurses' organisations and county doctors. One group of women researchers, of which I was a member, replied with a seventy-five-page document which pulled the risk system to pieces and made suggestions for new guidelines. The group consisted of five women (with fifteen children between us): two midwives, one doctor, one sociologist and one psychologist. Our report concluded that,

> The basis of any guidelines must be that pregnancy, birth and the postpartum period involves natural biological and psychological processes which are influenced by the culture that they exist in. If births are going to improve, they should not be taken out of and away from society and made into a medical issue. Even in industrial society, birth should be a part of the cultural basis of that society; this is unfortunately not the case. We must understand birth in its simplicity, as something that is part of being human.

In 1985 the final version of the perinatal guidelines was given out; these were immediately used as the basis for new birth plans in each county. They were unique in that they included nothing on risk groups. The introduction to the guidelines states, 'The perinatal period is a normal period of a family's life. The woman, her family and close friends should be central. The midwife, doctors and any other staff are there only to support the woman and her family.' The emphasis is placed on health and non-invasive care. The Board of Health, which was ultimately responsible for the guidelines, was awarded the annual prize from the large consumer organisation Parents and Birth.

It is in this framework that the midwife works today. What is her role?

DURING THE PREGNANCY

When a woman thinks she is pregnant she will usually have a pregnancy test done at a pharmacy. If if is positive she will see her own GP. The GP will examine her and discuss how she feels and the preferred place of birth. The GP will send reports to the closest midwife centre and hospital where she might want to give birth. When she is twelve weeks pregnant, the woman will see a midwife who, from that time on, will be the main professional attending the woman during her pregnancy. Together they plan how many antenatal visits there should be, and what form these should take. Generally a woman will visit her midwife six to eight times during the course of her pregnancy. The woman will see her GP again twice and has the option of visiting an obstetrician at the nearest hospital. The midwife spends fifteen to twenty minutes with her on each visit; it is not enough time, particularly as most of the visit is taken up with clinical matters. Certainly, if there is a need to talk, the midwife will make time, but one wonders how far the woman will feel at ease and able to talk when she knows that there are people waiting outside.

In a few places group consultations are held as part of projects. This allows more time as well as using the resources of the other pregnant women. A midwife will normally see between ten and twenty-five women in consultation during a day. She can refer to a doctor or perform ultrasound screening if necessary. Another important part of the midwives' antenatal work is the antenatal classes which take place in most hospitals or midwife centres and are usually taken by the midwives during their working hours. (Unfortunately this is not always the case and antenatal classes are the first things to be cut when there is a shortage of money or midwives.) An antenatal programme usually consists of six to eight lessons, each lasting two hours; sometimes the lessons are combined with one hour of physiotherapy. Several classes are open to partners as well.

DURING BIRTH

Whether a woman is having her baby at home or in a hospital, she will contact the local hospital when she goes into labour. There is always a midwife on call for home births. It is the midwife who assesses the situation, either in hospital or at home, and decides if and when to call a doctor.

During the labour and birth the midwife will stay with the woman, comforting her and giving her as much support as she needs. When the time comes the midwife helps the woman to give birth in the position she feels most relaxed in. Sometimes it is on a beanbag on the floor, and sometimes it is on all fours on the bed or supported by her partner who sits behind her. Sometimes there will be a doctor present at birth, but this usually happens only with a student doctor who is there for the experience. The midwife performs an episiotomy if necessary and sutures this as well as any tear. She can also perform a pudendal block if necessary. She examines the baby an hour or so after it is born (not immediately, as the baby and parents are left by themselves just after the birth). In hospital, the woman stays in the delivery ward for two hours after the birth. The midwife takes care of her and her baby, and completes the necessary paperwork. If the birth has taken place at home, the midwife usually stays for two or three hours afterwards.

THE PERIOD FOLLOWING THE BIRTH

Danish midwives do very little in the postnatal period. In most areas, time is allocated during their waking hours for postnatal visits both in the ward and in the home. Although postnatal visits work well in some areas of Denmark, in other areas, especially Copenhagen, they don't work. Usually the midwife who attended the birth will visit the woman whilst she is on the ward, and the antenatal midwife will go to the home to see her there. If it is a home birth or if the woman goes home just after the birth, both visits will take place in the home and will alternate with visits from the health visitor.

In one hospital in Copenhagen there is an ABC-clinic (alternative birth centre) with between 300 and 400 births each year.

The clinic is run only by midwives, who take care both of women giving birth and of women who stay there after the birth. There is very little intervention, and only women with routine pregnancies can give birth there. If anything happens during the birth the woman is transferred to the special unit in the same building. The clinic, although extremely popular with women and their families, has only just been able to survive, as the politicians claim that it is too expensive.

THE POPULARITY OF MIDWIFE CARE

Danish women like their midwives. There is a long tradition of good, solid midwifery care, and it is absolutely out of the question that GPs should take over. The obstetricians claim that they do not want to take over the routine births but sometimes the midwives, the women and the obstetricians have different ideas of what a routine pregnancy and birth is. In 1984 the Danish Institute of Epidemiology conducted a large survey to find out how women liked the perinatal services, on behalf of the Minister of Interior and as background for the new guidelines mentioned earlier. All women who gave birth in May 1984 were sent a twenty-eight-page questionnaire about six to eight weeks after they had given birth. Almost 4,000 women answered – a response rate of 81 per cent. The survey revealed the following.

During pregnancy, women preferred to get advice from the midwife. For various reasons women felt that they were able to discuss more issues with the midwife than with their own GP, issues like home delivery, where to get information about place of birth, consumer groups, their own economic situation and antenatal classes. Most women (92 per cent) felt that there needed to be at least twenty-five minutes set aside for each antenatal visit; this was sufficient time to get enough information and answers to their questions. Two-thirds (66 per cent) of the women felt that it would have been good to stay in touch with their midwife after the birth, and 80 per cent of those who had given birth at home felt it was important to know their midwife. Only 25 per cent of the women actually had a midwife whom they already knew or had met once or twice beforehand. More of these women said that they had had a good birth experience than did those who did not know their midwife. The majority of women questioned were in favour of postpartum visits, and yet only 10 per cent of those who live in Copenhagen are visited by a midwife at home, whilst women in Jutland all receive visits.

One of the women who answered the questionnaire said, 'My last birth has been a very positive experience, for which I feel I can thank my midwife. The important thing for me during the pregnancy was that I did not have to have the same midwife as I had the first time. I wish that one could know one's own midwife, but I guess that is impossible.' Another woman felt,

'Even when you plan to give birth in a hospital, you still need to know your midwife throughout the pregnancy and birth. I had five different midwives when I was in labour. The last one came just before I was going to push. The new midwife started by saying, "Now you turn on your back. I am giving the orders here and if you don't like it, you should have had a home birth." I wanted her to go away, but I suddenly became a patient and not a birthing woman. I think that the capacity of the midwifery profession should be large enough to allow every woman to choose a midwife who she feels confident with, who would follow her pregnancy and birth. A birth is a sexual event and what woman would go to bed with a man she has no confidence in?'

We know little about the midwives' feelings towards their work. We can get at least a sense of it from a questionnaire survey conducted in 1985 by four cultural sociology students. They interviewed fifty midwives from all over the country asking them how the introduction of technologies such as ultrasound, cardiography and amniocentesis had affected their jobs. One respondent said,

'It seems that the technology that is introduced to the perinatal area influences the organisation of midwives' work, partly because it leads to greater medical control with the births and with the midwifery work itself, as it causes a reduction in the midwives' work area. The technology results centralisation of pregnancy, birth and postpartum care in hospital units, where some of the functions of the midwives are taken over by the staff in the hospitals. And midwifery often loses its basic creative touch, because the traditional knowledge and habits of midwifery are pushed out in favour of tests and machines; consequently the midwife loses her independence in the work.'

But not all of the midwives shared this attitude towards the use of technology. A third of those interviewed were critical of cardiography, but most of the others used it in their daily work; 60 per cent of them thought that ultrasound scanning was overused. Generally, the more influence they could exert over when to use technology, the happier they felt about it.

Midwives all over Denmark are discussing their situation. We know that we must become more visible, ask questions, believe in our own feelings, and work closely together with the parents. And, most of all, we recognise the importance of midwife education.

THE EDUCATION OF MIDWIVES

The Danish midwifery school was founded in 1787, and in 1987 Danish midwives celebrated their 200th official anniversary. Before the school opened, older midwives taught younger midwives, a tradition that continued in rural areas well into the nineteenth century. The school was first part of a hospital, where unmarried women could give birth free of charge and possibly leave behind their babies. The mortality rate was high: in 1839, 57 per cent of these women died during birth or postpartum.

Today there are two midwifery schools in Denmark, one in Copenhagen and one in Aalborg, Jutland. Each year forty students start the training and midwifery has become one of the most difficult educational programmes to get into. This means that the midwifery students who are accepted already have other medical training, both theoretical and practical, and/or very high grades from high school. The students are bright and outspoken, with strong opinions, and they are frequently quite critical of high-tech births. Both midwifery schools offer direct-entry three-year programmes with theoretical periods in school and practical periods working in clinics. The first year is spent at the university hospital, where women with special needs referred from all over Denmark mix with women expecting normal births. The next two years of the student's training take place in large hospitals, except for a short period of five weeks when they can go anywhere in Denmark. Some of the students choose small midwife centres where there 'are no machines'; others will work in hospitals. Very few midwives drop out. More than 90 per cent use their training and only stop working on retirement.

Usually there are a few nurses on the courses and they can complete the training in two years. This has generated a great deal of discussion recently about midwife training. Should midwifery education be built on nursing education or not? At the moment, the feeling is that it should not. Because both the training and professional practice of midwives are regarded as health-promoting activities midwifery is not a curing profession, and cannot be seen as supplementary to nursing.

THE DANISH ASSOCIATION OF MIDWIVES

Danish midwives are organised in a small but energetic organisation, the Danish Association of Midwives. There are 1,200 midwives altogether, of whom 700 are working full-time and 200 part-time; the rest either have teaching positions or are retired. Each county has its own board, consisting only of midwives. These groups meet once a month and all the midwives in each county meet every second month. Representatives from each county meet six times a year in a big group assembly. Some counties are very active with regular discussion days where all kinds of themes are discussed and presented, such as the role of the midwife in family planning, midwives and technology, and so on. There are other subcommittees directly under the secretariat, such as the education committee, the research and development committee, and the technology committee. These groups are active and arrange a number of courses for the midwives. Five years ago the Association employed an educational consultant and since then there have been a number of very good and exciting courses. Most Danish midwives have been on one or other of these courses; apart from providing additional knowledge, the courses give them a very important chance to meet and talk. The Association also arranges 'theme days' on different 'hot' issues like alternative pain relief, ultrasound, and the midwife's role in ultrasound. And most recently we have had research and development days to encourage midwives to do research. Some of the inspiration for the courses comes from the Radical Midwives and the Active Birth Movement. As we are a small association we must avoid dividing up into smaller fractions and so far this has been possible.

The Association has a monthly journal, *Journal for Midwives*, with a full-time editor, which is a very important means of communication between the midwives. Over the last years it has been interesting to see how many more of the articles are written by midwives about midwifery, rather than by doctors.

HOW WE COMMUNICATE WITH OTHERS

Midwives have a tendency to believe that they have a job for which there will always be a demand. As a result we have not felt it necessary to participate in the public debate and we do not see ourselves as political persons. This is probably just as much a 'women's issue' as a 'midwife issue'. We do our jobs, take care of our families, are a bit overworked because of the long shift hours and have no time left for political work.

The Association of Midwives is, of course, represented in the government group that deals with legislation concerning midwifery and perinatal services, but the 'ordinary' midwife is seldom vocal in public. A postgraduate course could be seen as a way to make ourselves more competitive with other professionals in the medical world. We do have the advantage that we are from a country with profound democratic traditions without a strict hierarchical system. Ours is not a society which constrains people with energy and good ideas.

Midwives have always been, and still are, greatly respected in the community. We do not make ourselves very conspicuous although we know we should. We are at the moment trying to find a good way to communicate with the obstetricians. We have formed a midwife-obstetrician forum where we meet and discuss common interests, and we try especially to sort out the misconceptions each group has of the other. Midwives generally feel a great solidarity with women and families, and many Danish midwives are members of the large consumer organisation Parents and Childbirth. This organisation is fifteen years old and has an important role in humanising the perinatal services in Denmark.

OUR HOPES AND DREAMS OF THE FUTURE

Let us close our eyes and imagine what the perinatal and midwifery future will be in Denmark. By the year 2000 midwives will work in small groups of three and four. They will work closely together in a multidisciplinary group consisting of consumers, health visitors, GPs, home-visiting nurses, district psychologists and social workers. The group will work within the primary health group and cover a smaller geographical area. Seminars and meetings will be held between the different primary and secondary health groups, with built-in evaluation systems which will ensure that health promotion work is done. All health workers must work on their own fitness, both physical and psychological, as their own good health is essential to their work. The midwives will operate from small clinics where all the other health workers will be based. The midwives will work in pairs and have group consultations with three to four couples or single woman. There will also be the possibility for talking alone with the midwife. Antenatal classes as such will not exist. Instead of classes, there will be self-help groups, where the emphasis is put on working with expectations, concepts of oneself, relationships, and with one's own birth experience. Birth films will not be shown any more and instead one will work therapeutically with one's own birth and the coming birth. The self-help groups will be the basis for the networks and will be formed so that the participants live close to one another. Slowly a new understanding of pregnancy, birth and the period after birth will emerge. This was given impetus in 1985 when guidelines were developed for perinatal care. The birth is not so central any more. The pregnancy and the care are now just as important. The midwives have gained a new understanding of their work now that they have the opportunity to give continuity of care. This, combined with working in a dynamic, multidisciplinary group with possibilities for their own development, has given them new insights.

There has been a steady rise in home births and 'domino' births and now the proportion of these are steady at 15 to 20 per cent. No birth unit has more than 800 births per year. The midwives feel that they make the initial relationship with the primary health group, and that has opened up the hospitals. The specialists have more time and they work as peripatetic consultants wherever they are needed. There are developmental groups that look at routines and treatment methods and assess them physically, psychologically, ethically and scientifically. The birth units are small, where the women both give birth and stay in some days afterwards with the same staff around them. The midwives look after both the birthing and the postpartum women. New research and birth knowledge has meant that very little medicine is used. The woman's endorphins usually work very well, as the surroundings support the family at the birth in all possible ways. Allergy research shows that methergin and oxytoxic should not be used. The men whose children are born in these units are very much closer to the baby; it has now been shown that, especially in the first days, the development of father-infant bonding is very strong. Often the father stays in the hospital for the whole period, if the birth takes place there. (Some feminists claim that the men are taking over the children from the moment of birth.)

The midwives clearly have their own identity in the local community and at the same time they are esteemed members of the multidisciplinary health group that not only works with pregnant and birthing women, but also considers all the factors in society that are important for the local community. They teach at the schools and give counselling on all reproduction matters. Cost-benefit analyses, or rather technological assessments, are continually undertaken, which include consideration of psychological factors for both clients and practitioners. When the midwives were assessed, it was found that they were working on bringing out the resources in the families who were having a baby, and they had the knowledge and skills to support the families when resources were scarce. The midwife is back in the limelight, developing and working as a true team member within the health group.

But before we get there. . . .

WHAT IS TO BE DONE?

A report on birth, midwives, parents and technology states,

> It is our impression that the midwife could disappear as an independent professional in a perinatal system where the dominant thinking is the risk approach. We are seeing the midwife squeezed between the obstetrician and the pregnant woman. She is going to work together with both. It looks as if the midwives' group has difficulties in standing up to the doctors' group. (Mette Höyen Andersen and Ruth Sillemann, 1985).

But a Danish midwife, and teacher, Inge Guilbert, who is very vocal about perinatal issues, told me,

> 'I think it important that midwives are aware of new developments in the perinatal field. Although it is important to reduce perinatal mortality, we must use our profession so that this happens with the help of the midwives' traditional methods: humanity, alertness, patience, tolerance and understanding. We must use all our clinical understanding and theoretical knowledge to assess the birthing woman's whole situation. Technology can be an important help, but it must never be the factor that is running a birth. It must be the task of the midwives in the consultant unit to change not only the physical surroundings, but also the psychological. The midwife must help and assist so that the birth (even in a consultant unit) becomes not an illness with a fast recovery, but a healthy and natural ending to a pregnancy and the beginning of a new human being's life. The midwives ought to guarantee that the birth will be treated as normal until the opposite is proved, and not allow what happens today, that the birth is complicated until with all kinds of methods you have proved that it is totally normal.'

The midwives also face pressure from the government, as scarcer resources have meant that the county midwives are being made redundant. This means that midwives have less influence at the decision-making level.

From this it is clear that there are three major obstacles for the continuation of midwifery as an independent profession: (1) lack of influence in important places; (2) doctors; (3) technology.

MIDWIVES AND DOCTORS

A report on midwives and technology (Gammeltoft *et al.*, 1985) describes the conflict between midwives and doctors as follows.

As the set of norms that the midwives and the obstetricians have is very different, the midwives are in a dilemma. The reasons why it is the midwives and not the doctors who have a hard time are:

(1) The most prominent social values in society and in the health system legitimise the set of norms held by doctors.

(2) Doctors have more power because of their higher status. This means that doctors as a profession, and the health system in general, are putting great pressure on the midwifery group and their status in society. Furthermore, there is also pressure on the midwife group from doctors as well as other professions in the health sector, because of their interest in well-being. There is less money given to the health sector by the government and there is growing unemployment. Therefore other professions have a growing interest in taking over some of the midwives' work areas. The result of this is that the midwives are in a crisis. Technological values confront humanistic values. The midwives who see this become very interested in fighting for the survival of midwifery.

MIDWIVES AND TECHNOLOGY

What has happened to midwives after technology was introduced in the mid-1970s? Just as the 'risk' approach becomes self-fulfilling, so too does the introduction of technology. This self-fulfilling process takes place on the basis of a change in the set of norms and consciousness in the users of the system as well as in the health personnel, and that includes midwives. Eli Heiberg Endresen, a Norwegian physiotherapist and anthropologist, writes about this:

When technology is used more it creates a gradual change of consciousness both within the personnel and in their clients. After a while you take the resources for granted and the advanced technology becomes routine. At births today we see how ultrasound and cardiography try to be a routine, not only in special situations but also in ordinary healthy situations – just to be sure. When a society uses sophisticated technology, changes are going to be made on many levels. The concrete reality and the social practice change and a greater awareness takes place amongst people using the technology. This change leads to dependence on the technology. We get the impression of endless possibilities for saving lives, if only the resources were large enough. The techniques very quickly become necessary and wanted in people's minds because who dares to say now that it is impossible. Technology has this implicit ability to secure its own growth – and our dependency.

So what was said earlier about the opposing points of view of those running the health system and midwives is no longer accurate. Midwives themselves are changing because of the technology. Pressure like this on the midwives' own perception of pregnancy and birth, both because of changes in the midwives' themselves (which they probably are not aware of) and because of the changes among the women, could lead to a falling apart of the centre for the midwives groups' own social values.

WHERE ARE WE GOING?

In this situation of being pressurised from three sides, being confused about our own role in the rapidly changing perinatal scene, being overworked and not very vocal about our situation, what is likely to happen? Either we shall disappear, or stay but as shadows of ourselves, with no influence and with no power at the decision-making level or in our daily work. Or something else can happen. In Gammeltoft *et al.*'s report on midwives and birth technology, the authors make the following suggestions.

But the midwives can do something else. Instead of disappearing they can go in another direction. The conflict can lead to a holding-on to the midwives' social values and cultural orientation. Midwives could join together and fight for a solution to keeping and spreading their own social values. To do this they need to work collectively and to have the opportunity to put forward their future goals. There is a need for an organisational structure that can tie the different parts of the movement together into a cohesive group. These changes could be channelled through the Danish Association of Midwives.

We think that is the way we are going. In 1983 a conference on birth was held in the World Health Organisation's buildings in Copenhagen, supported by WHO and arranged by the Danish Association of Midwives. A quarter of all Danish midwives were there, together with representatives from other related health organisations. This was somehow a turning point. We realised for the first time that we had a common goal: to support women and their families in having a good birth experience, that would give the newborn and the family the best start possible with one another. After the conference we celebrated all night, knowing in our hearts that we would never give up, and feeling extremely grateful that we were midwives and deeply responsible for the future of our profession.

REFERENCES

Andersen, Mette Höyen, and Silleman, Ruth, *Ammestuesnak*, RUC, 1985.

Gammeltoft, T., Hansen, L.L., Molholm, M.B. and Poulsen, J., *Midwives and Birth Technology: Where Are They Going?*, Cultural Social Institute, Copenhagen, 1985.

Journal for Midwives, no. 3, March 1987.

Kamper-Jörgensen, Finn, Madsen Mette, Torben, Sörensen K., Roepstorff, Christian, Bjerregaard, Peter, *Pregnancy, Birth, and Choice of Birth Place*, DIKE, 1985.

'The status of midwives through time', by students from the Danish midwifery school, Copenhagen, 1967, unpublished.

Anne Margrete Berg *et al.* (eds), *Womenfolk, no. I: A History of Denmark from 1600 to 1980*, Gyldendal, 1984.

INTRODUCTION

FRANCE

In France care in pregnancy is usually under the control of the obstetrician rather than the midwife, but there are different combinations including some GP care and a shared care system similar to that in Britain, in which responsibility is divided between the GP and the staff of a maternity unit. Midwives are more involved during labour than in pregnancy, though they do only 39 per cent of all normal deliveries in hospital, compared with 100 per cent in Sweden and Finland and 95 per cent in Norway. Routine shaving is still often practised and a fixed posture for delivery may be obligatory, except in advanced units where 'alternative' childbirth is practised, and in home births, for which there is now a growing demand.[1]

As in many other countries, the stand taken by independent midwives who do home births is important for the profession as a whole, and for the humanisation of childbirth. Only when midwives can work outside the hospital system, and resist being sucked into hierarchically organised teams under the direction of an obstetrician, can they practise fully the profession for which they are trained. And only in this way can a real personal relationship be guaranteed between the midwife and the woman and her family throughout pregnancy, birth and the postnatal period. The existence of a strong independent midwifery is empowering for *all* midwives.

NOTE

1 Phaff, J.M.L. (ed.), *Perinatal Health Services in Europe* (World Health Organisation), Croom Helm, 1986.

THE MIDWIFE IN FRANCE

HAMMANI FARIDA

(translated by Madeleine Ruehl for Material Word Ltd*)

'It was natural that a mother who had given birth should offer her advice and assistance to inexperienced women. Once this help had been repeated several times, it was also natural that people had faith in her and called upon her. That is how the first midwife came into being.' (*Siebolt*)

Wise woman, healer, witch, obstetrician, 'doctor with limited responsibilities', in a word *sage-femme*, no less. . . .

Where does it begin, this long complicity between women and midwives, and where does it end? Through the course of the centuries and the vicissitudes of politics and religion, the French midwife, central pillar of maternity until the thirteenth century, was by turns burnt as a 'witch' under the inquisition and then rehabilitated by the church, and she was caught in the cross-fire in the war between the new physicians and the barber-surgeons from the sixteenth to the eighteenth centuries. She also created the first schools of obstetrical training, with Mme du Coudray's school founded in 1757 and Mme La Chapelle's around 1800, but nevertheless, the midwife suffered the effects of unfair laws, in particular the 1892 law which weakened her position.

Finally, in 1945 the profession suffered a great setback when the establishment locked up the French midwife in hospitals and clinics, allowing her, in effect, only an auxiliary medical role. This could have been a death blow. And yet now, as before, the French midwife survives and remains the woman with technical

---

* Translator's note: the term '*libéral*' has been translated throughout as 'independent'.

expertise, as well as an accomplice and friend, who has the privilege of accompanying women in labour. Ever more active in the technical field – her right to prescribe and administer treatment has increased at a faster rate over the past four years than in the previous twenty – her influence grows daily with the authorities, thanks to the various associations that represent her.

And it remains the case that in France all women are accompanied by a midwife during childbirth.

1900–1945

In 1892 a law authorising physicians and health officers, as well as midwives, to practice obstetrics brought about a further decline in the profession of midwifery. Indeed, not only was the study of medicine becoming more structured at that time, but also women were prevented from entering the medical profession.

On the other hand, a split-level training in midwifery was allowed to emerge, producing, in broad terms, first-class midwives trained in two years at the schools that existed, and second-class midwives recruited at a level only just equivalent to that of the school certificates. There were more second-class midwives, of course, and this imbalance contributed to the profession's reputation for obscurantism, a reputation which was skilfully engineered by the medical profession. At the same time, the birth rate was falling, and midwives did not have access to any professional organ of information, still less to any body which might defend their rights. (The first association of midwives in France was not created until 1913.) The number of obstetricians increased, even though it was possible for one writer to say that 'many pupils became doctors without having examined a woman or been present at a birth. This seems horrendous, but it is the case.' As a consequence of this veritable negation of our profession, in 1916 Mlle Mosse, chief midwife of the Paris maternity unit, deplored the independent midwives' disastrous situation:

At the moment, our profession is going through a crisis, and to set oneself up as a midwife does not mean to say that one can find any work. Not only has the number of births diminished since 1915, but the number dealt with by hospitals is proportionately higher than in peacetime. The reports of some of our colleagues lead to the conclusion that the situation is as sad as it is widespread.

An Act passed in 1916 narrowed down midwifery qualifications to a single diploma and marked a step forward in the history of the profession: 'While the auxiliary midwives may have brought dishonour to the profession, there are others whose life of self-denial, or rectitude in the face of poverty . . . can arouse only admiration, and they are by far the greatest number' (Pr BAR, 1916).

Midwives at this time must have been wonderful women, on the road night and day, working for a pittance, attacked on every side by the medical profession, the law and the hospitals which insidiously robbed them of their clientele. So who are they, then, these 'unworthy' midwives? Could they be these women, these midwives, moved by the distress of one of their patients at the announcement of her eighth or tenth pregnancy, or perhaps of an 'illegitimate' pregnancy, at a time when contraception didn't even exist who in the light of their own conscience performed abortions? Were they not women first and foremost, in their hearts and bodies? Today, contraception is legalised and widespread, and hundreds of abortions are performed in France every day. Abortionists ('angel-makers'), my sisters, I salute you as benefactors of suffering humanity.

All of these problems facing the midwife were exacerbated in the cities. In the countryside, the reproduction of the species remained an exclusively female province. As one midwife in the Ardèche, Mlle B. recalled,

'Because at that time it was customary to give birth in one's own bed, progress in the field of medicine had not yet claimed the right to interfere with the act of childbirth. This fear of childbirth, this panic which now poisons our existence, did not then exist. In those days, if a midwife's client chose to give birth with her help, but in a maternity ward, it was not so much as a result of medical advice as through not having the right conditions or support from those around her. Women only gave birth outside the home if they did not have a family, neighbours or a husband capable of looking after them and their babies.'

A midwife working as an independent practitioner in maternity wards, whether private or public, was then 'in control of the process and did not have to answer to anyone else. She supervised the birth, looked after the newborn child, and came on the following days to take care of the mother and keep an eye on the child, exactly as she would have done in a private house.' Before 1945, some private hospitals and clinics did exist, but it was the independent activity of the practitioners in the area which guaranteed their functioning. Certain establishments, annexed to a school of midwifery or a faculty of medicine, granted some midwives the status of salaried employees but it was more in their capacity as teachers in the school than in their capacity as practitioners. The hospital was, above all, for unmarried mothers. Mlle B. remembers,

'When these creatures, having no other choice, ended up confessing to their mothers that they were going to have a baby, only too often the mother, by way of reprisal, simply packed the guilty girl off to hospital. When an unknown, pregnant girl turned up at the gates of the maternity hospital, the nun in charge urgently phoned around the district trying to find a practitioner. Meanwhile, the woman, in labour all this time, completely alone, losing fluid and blood, racked by all the pains in the world, waited in a corner.'

So, with the hospitals reserved for the 'poor unfortunates', in a material or moral sense, the average French woman, with the help of a midwife she trusted and sometimes that of a family doctor too, gave birth at home, in her own environment, supported by family and friends.

What has happened to us, then, over the past forty years? Why has there been a frantic recourse to gynaecologists? Why this dread in the face of childbirth? This abdication of responsibility? This staggering, routine use of epidural injections? This rapid increase in Caesareans? What sort of humanity is there in this form of childbirth when women are put on a drip, monitored, tied to a delivery table, given epidural injections, and neverthe-less thank these new magicians in boots, masks and gloves who deliver them in complete safety? *Where are the midwives?*

1945: HOSPITAL-BASED MIDWIVES

The new social laws in force after the Liberation were based on good intentions. Why and how did they deliver an (almost) fatal blow to the midwifery profession? The right to social security benefits became more widespread . . . fine! Direct payment by insurers was introduced for women going into hospital to give birth . . . aha! . . . Not for those who wanted to stay at home! . . . One might have thought that the hospital, still operating as an open clinic, would have paid the independent midwife (several months late, of course, but that's no surprise). But open clinics in public hospitals gradually died out. And midwives worked in clinics and hospitals where they had to act under the orders of doctors.

Let us return to the words of Mlle B., the midwife in the Ardèche. This is how she described the situation after 1945.

'With the Liberation, new laws came into force which intro-duced social security, reformed the way maternity hospitals were run and considerably favoured hospital deliveries. In so doing, they struck a severe blow against the corporate body of independent midwives. Most of my colleagues were unable to hold out against the storm and abandoned the profession. But I am still here. Thirty-five years on, I'm still travelling around the mountains of the Ardèche and elsewhere, with my little black leather bag and my white apron. I am still going. I have had doors slammed in my face, as have my colleagues, but, for some unknown reason, other doors, great and splendid ones, have been opened to me, leading me off down paths along which I never expected to venture.'

The great strength of the 1945 and 1946 Acts is that they grouped together the many bodies involved in social insurance provision to wider sections of the population. It should also be said however that some steps had already been taken before 1945 to reimburse the costs of childbirth. From 1935 onwards, women who had paid their national insurance contributions and wives of men who were insured, had their doctor's and chemist's bills relating to pregnancy, childbirth and aftercare paid in full, as well as hospital bills where this applied. Before 1935, only a part of this expense had been reimbursed by the various different social insurance funds, as they had gradually been set up and had accepted, as part of their responsibilities, payments to cover the costs of childbirth.

The crucial innovation of the postwar period consisted neither in the fact that costs incurred in childbirth were reimbursed, nor even that they were paid in full. What profoundly changed our profession and, consequently, the normal circumstances of pregnancy and childbirth, was a marginal clause in the new Acts, which was apparently minor and innocuous. This clause stipulated that when birth took place in a public hospital the reimbursement procedure was simplified so that the mother had nothing at all to pay; the Social Security Department assumed responsibility for the costs and undertook to pay the hospital direct. In other words, while everything was free for women who agreed to go into hospital, those who insisted on giving birth at home not only had to pay fees to the doctor or midwife who attended the birth and looked after them during the following days, but also had to buy everything that the midwife might require from the chemist. Admittedly, the money spent would be refunded in full, but as in the prewar period, the mother had to make the initial payment herself.

Some mothers could be exempted from making this payment, even if they were giving birth at home. In this case they had to have recourse to the 'due authorisation in advance' system, which is still in force today. On the social security form, in place of the signature certifying that our fees have been properly paid, we write 'DAA'. This tells the social insurance fund that it must not reimburse the insured mother, but directly pay us, the midwives. Unfortunately, not all social security offices accept DAA, and those which do, only do so in exceptional circumstances, usually when the mother's income is particularly low. The public maternity hospital, on the other hand, has been absolutely free since the Liberation and takes all women, so long as they either pay national insurance contributions or are rightful claimants as dependants of an insured person.

It is easy to see how such a measure has contributed to making hospital births a standard feature of life. We independent midwives could have adapted to these developments if the reforms had stopped there, and if our right to practise on open wards in the public maternity hospitals had been maintained, since we are by no means averse to attending our clients there if that is where they wish to give birth. (If I still have a preference for home births, it is because of the spontaneous celebrations to which they give rise, and to which I am always so warmly invited.)

In 1945, on the recommendation of the Ministers of Justice, Public Health and Labour, the Vichy government placed the governing board of the Midwives' Association under the aegis of the French Association of Physicians. The aims of the French Association of Midwives are:

- to ensure that the principles of morality, integrity and dedication that are indispensable for the practice of medicine are maintained;
- to ensure the defence of the profession's honour and independence;
- to unite all the members of the profession with the aim of maintaining the high levels of morality and independence that are necessary for the full flowering of a liberal profession.

A doctor was made president of the board of the Association and, currently, the governing board of the Association of French Midwives comprises four doctors and five midwives. A referendum organised in 1982 by the *Les Dossiers de l'obstetrique* magazine showed that most French midwives did not want to see their Association disappear. However, all the midwives demanded that the president of the Association should be a midwife and that doctors should be involved only in a consultative capacity. In spite of the promises, we are still waiting.

Not all midwives agree that the Association should be kept in existence. Some even go so far as to refuse to pay their obligatory subscription, and find themselves charged with 'illegal practice of medicine' and sentenced to fines of more than 10,000 francs.

In France, some 200 midwives are currently attempting – most often on their own – to oppose the requirement that they belong to the Association. Some are doing so because they feel there is no longer any justification for the existence of professional associations and they only serve to maintain a medical system based on privilege, which is out of tune with the development of society and the needs of the population. Others oppose it because they think the Association in its current form does not meet the needs of practising midwives and it should be transformed. (*L'Impatient*, 1982, no. 101)

In 1949 a code of ethics was created governing the profession of midwifery. As Mme Jeannette Bessonart writes in *Le Lien et les masques*, 'You could be forgiven for having the impression there were no midwives in France before 1949, since at that stage there was no code and before September 1945, no Association!' But these two structures were simply a further means for doctors to gain control over experiences women had been sharing for many years. They were trying to take the unique relationship that had formed between the mother, her relatives and the independent midwife and keep it 'under observation'. Having an Association and an ethical code for midwives conceals the way in which we have been brought to heel under the authority of doctors whose intention is that we should become mere medical auxiliaries.

The first trade unions were formed among French midwives during the 1940s. These have recently been reorganised into two bodies with large memberships. They are the Organisation Nationale des Syndicats de Sages Femmes Françaises, which publishes a news magazine entitled *L'Officiel de la sage femme*, and the Union Nationale des Sages Femmes Françaises, both of which have their headquarters in Paris.

Over the years midwives, both within their organisations and as individuals, have sought to resist the ever-increasing pressure from a medical establishment which is constantly growing in size and is bolstered by an increasingly machine-orientated medicalisation of childbirth. Moreover, all the high-tech developments are sustained by media interest; the exceptional always makes better copy than the commonplace.

In 1982, an Act 'Concerning the Profession of Midwifery in France' came into force. Article L.374 states,

The activities falling within the profession of midwifery include the performance of procedures necessary for the diagnosis and supervision of pregnancy and psychoprophylactic preparation for childbirth, together with supervising and conducting the delivery and the provision of postnatal care of mother and child.

. . . It may also fall within the ambit of the midwife to participate in consultations on family planning matters.

. . . Midwives are authorised to prescribe diaphragms, caps and other barrier contraceptives. The first fitting of a diaphragm or cap must be carried out by a doctor or a midwife.

There follows a long list of the medicines which a midwife is allowed to prescribe, together with a list of the physical and radiological examinations she may need to carry out either for the mother or the child in the course of a normal pregnancy or delivery. It would take too long to list all these here. Suffice it to say that the French midwife, unlike many of her colleagues in the EEC, is, by her rights of prescription and treatment, an autonomous practitioner in her specialist field, recognised by French law as belonging to one of the three medical professions (the other two being doctors and dental surgeons).

THE SITUATION OF FRENCH MIDWIVES TODAY

In 1983 and 1984, *Les Dossiers de l'obstetrique*, a magazine of medical and professional information for midwives, alerted by rumours of unemployment within the profession, carried out a survey on the employment situation among midwives. This revealed that many small maternity units, both public and private, were being closed down. Midwives were out of work and receiving varying levels of unemployment benefit. Some, who had formerly held posts of great responsibility, had been relegated to a nursing role. In the private clinics, there were now cases of employers telling midwives who demanded better working conditions or rates of pay that if they were not happy they could leave: 'There are ten people waiting to take your job!' Previously, the midwife had been seen as a rare and precious

Table 1a Development of the professions of midwife, gynaecological and obstetric specialist and general practitioner, measured by number of registered practitioners on 1 January 1974, 1978, and 1983.

| | Independent activity | | | Salaried activity | | | Total | | |
	1974	1978	1983	1974	1978	1983	1974	1978	1983
Midwives	2,345	2,145*	1,477*	6,029	6,313	7,183	8,374	8,458 (a)	8,660
Specialists in gynaecology* and obstetrics	1,523	2,007	2,819	227	450	870	1,750	2,457	3,689
General practitioners	31,400	39.262	48,622	14,795	18,453	22,168	46,195	57,715	70,790 (e)

Table 1b Medical practitioners by profession on 1 January 1974 and 1983

	1974	1983
Total		
Doctors	73,552	118,000 (e)
Dental surgeons	23,882	33,048
Pharmacists	18,470	43,662
Midwives	8,374	8,660

Source: CNAMS.
* This covers all the specialists in gynaecology, gynaecology and obstetrics, and obstetrics.
(a)=adjusted   (e)=estimate

person, and treated as such. The figures in Table 1 speak for themselves. They show that, between 1974 and 1983,

- midwives have seen their numbers increase by 286, while in the same period, doctors specialising in obstetrics have increased by 1,939;
- the number of general practitioners has almost doubled in this period; I would remind the reader that every doctor in France has the right to deliver babies;
- the number of independent midwives has been halved in nine years, whilst the number of specialists in obstetrics has almost doubled.

The survey also provides evidence relating to midwives' employment (or unemployment) conditions:

- the posts currently occupied lack security;
  - young midwives find it increasingly difficult to get official posts;
- there is seasonal unemployment, which seems to have become accepted as normal;
- midwives work very flexible hours, making it possible to avoid creating jobs;
- midwives work in paramedical professions to survive;
- midwives take little maternity leave or leave of absence.

In short, the whole spectrum of midwives' working conditions is deteriorating. And, as Mme A. Delayen, chief ward-sister at Aulnay-sous-Bois says, 'It seems important to realise that in future, midwives will have to adopt a policy of keeping their eyes and ears open, and telling the world what is happening.'

What is the position of independent midwives? This is the view of Mme Joelle Le Goff, a midwife at Millau:

'There are currently around 9,000 midwives working in France, of whom 1,250 are independent. This latter figure is relatively high, but it might be of interest to take a closer look at the actual activities of those concerned.

The majority of these midwives provide nursing care, sometimes complementing this with antenatal work, either alone or in collaboration with medical practitioners (most often GPs or gynaecologists) or private clinics. Others conduct antenatal courses at swimming baths. Lastly, there are those who visit women with high-risk pregnancies at their homes, either working with gynaecologists who do not make home visits themselves or at the request of Public Health Department centres or hospitals.

Very few independent midwives have the opportunity of doing deliveries – fifty or perhaps a hundred at the outside. Very few have the means to practise their profession in all its aspects, that is, to monitor pregnancies, to prepare women for birth and attend the delivery. This is a great pity, and a very sad situation.'

There are and always will be women who prefer treatment and antenatal care from a midwife. Yet most have no idea that independent midwives still exist. In spite of the torrent of articles and programmes aimed at future parents, the media never mention the existence of independent midwives. In fact they do not mention midwives at all. Journalists manage to write about childbirth quite happily without referring to our profession. Yet of the 800,000 births which occur each year in France most are carried out or, at least, attended by midwives.

The enormous barrage of publicity surrounding childbirth encourages women to go to obstetricians and to hospitals. Today the maternity wards in public hospitals are closed to midwives and the private clinics which allow them in to deliver their clients' babies are few and far between. This is a central problem for the independent midwife. There remains the alternative of home delivery, which many of us practise. But the situation is difficult and commitment is needed to establish oneself in the 1980s.

In our day-to-day existence independent midwives face opposition from the social security and from other health professionals: pharmacists, radiologists, gynaecologists and, sometimes, our own colleagues in midwifery who are surprised by the degree of autonomy independent midwives enjoy and are misinformed about our true professional skills.

I should not paint an even darker picture of an already gloomy situation: independent practice does represent a form of freedom that is of real value.

THE WAR OF WORDS AND THE WAR OF NERVES

23 January 1986, Decree no. 86.124, Ethical Code of Midwives. The Prime Minister and Council of State decree:

Article 25: *The midwife is authorised to practise ultrasound scanning in the context of supervision of pregnancy, etc.*

MEDICINE'S ARISTOCRATS RECOIL IN HORROR!!!

From *Le Quotidien du médécin*, (*The Doctor's Daily*)

So as to ensure that scanning during pregnancy remains a medical act the Federation of Specialist Medical Practitioners issued a statement calling for the decree authorising midwives to perform this type of examination to be revoked. They reasoned that scanning requires supervision by a doctor, 'given the serious difficulties of interpretation in pathological cases', and complained that 'separating off the intellectual aspect from this technical operation marks the beginning of an undermedicalisation which would bring about a lowering of the care and standards of safety to which mothers-to-be are entitled'.

In 1982, with the new equal opportunities employment legislation, a *man* entered the profession! This led to discussions in the Councils of State and even to competitions in serious medical journals to determine what the poor young man's title would be. It was suggested that the name of the whole profession should be changed. Would we become the *maieuticians* or *periobstetricians* of tomorrow? Happily midwives were there with a solution. In France, we have women on industrial tribunals who are called '*prud'hommes*', so we would have men called '*sages femmes*' ('midwives'). The matter was settled.

At the National Conference of Midwives held in 1984, student midwives declared,

> Within the framework of the theme of this conference, 'what kind of childbirth in the future?', and given the preliminary comments made by the various roundtable discussion groups, it is clear to the student midwives here that the schools of midwifery no longer provide training adequate to meet present demands.
>
> In particular, our hypermedicalised and largely technical studies neglect the human aspect touched upon over the last few days, and leave little room for any broadening of the mind. In this respect, indeed, they work against it.
>
> As the midwives in charge of these future births, we declare that a total rethinking of our course of studies, both in its form and content, is a matter of urgency, and in this we count on the support of clients and members of the profession.

By 1985 midwifery training was extended to four years, and importance is now placed on psychology courses and learning about different methods of preparing for birth, giving the students a broader concept of their profession by offering more varied course options. From now on, the training will not be designed exclusively for hospital-based midwives. Several schools of midwifery, including the Ecole Nationale de Cadres, are for the first time inviting independent midwives to come and tell students how they work.

At the Les Entretiens de Bichat Conference in 1985 in Paris Professor Malinas, an eminent figure in French obstetrics, sounded an alarm bell by calling attention to the high rate of caesareans in France (20–40 per cent of births depending on the area) and confirmed that 'in certain places, women only have a chance to give birth naturally when there hasn't been time to call out what is pompously referred to as the "obstetric team"' (*Le Monde*, 18 October 1985). Later that year the National Federation of Patients' Associations was formed. It asserted that a woman should be cared for in labour by, and give birth with the help of, the practitioner of her choice, preferably the one who has supervised her pregnancy and prepared her for the birth. Under pressure from patients, by 1986 the media were showing overwhelming support for midwives: *Parents* magazine announced, 'Several thousand of you have responded to our survey of midwives and the exceptional interest shown in your replies has persuaded us to give an especially broad scope to the debate which we have decided to organise.' (broadcast on one of France's main TV channels, TF1). *Parents* continued,

One observation emerges right away: women think that midwives are wonderful! Ninety-two per cent of them find midwives gentle, warm and competent, 60 per cent think that midwives are qualified to prescribe and supervise contraception, 80 per cent agree that they should carry out scans, and that the use of forceps when necessary should fall within their domain (a right which midwives have never demanded). And because most women associate midwives with the act of giving birth, 75 per cent think that midwives should not carry out abortions (which midwives have not demanded either).

Although there are not enough of them to replace their colleagues who are going into retirement, midwives all over France are setting themselves up independently and are working.

Business is so good that after five years or so, most have to find someone to serve as a locum on a regular basis, or form a partnership with a colleague. How many doctors nowadays can say as much, especially in the big cities?

In March 1987 independent midwives compiled their own statistics for the first time and submitted these to the Ministry of Health. The figures show that, taking both kinds of practice together (approximately 51 per cent are home births and 49 per cent take place in hospital), only 4.8 per cent of births attended by independent midwives are caesareans, while the national average is 11 per cent. Independent midwives argue that the social security system benefits from these savings, as does the French taxpayer; at a time when the government is considering abolishing the social security system if it falls into financial ruin, such an argument carries some weight. The government is demanding the reopening of the private sector in public maternity hospitals for midwives only, since they have proved their public usefulness.

Owing to the closure of numerous small maternity hospitals (those dealing with fewer than 200 births each year), women all over France are being persuaded that for their own safety they should give birth in the 'super' maternity hospitals. These may be situated 30, 40 even 70 kilometres from their homes. When you have given birth in a car, you understand what the word 'safety' means. When you have entrusted your body to complete strangers, when you have been subjected to staff making some thirty-six invasions into your body every day (figures compiled at the ADASSA clinic in Strasbourg, but applicable to any maternity ward in France), you begin to understand the meaning of the words 'technical' and 'intimacy'.

The combination of the closure of small maternity units, which causes unemployment among midwives and leads women to refuse to go so far from home to give birth, and the collapse of the social security system all militates in favour of a revival of our profession. If the social security system survives, as all of us in France hope it will, and due regard is taken to the figures we have drawn up, it should be adapted to enhance and no longer to hinder the work of midwives. And we midwives, women and sisters of women giving birth, bear witness with commitment and a sense of reverence, to the role which everyone has been trying to wrest from us for centuries; we have been privileged to be present since the dawn of time at the birth of life. We midwives, have we not been through the most tempestuous of storms?

REFERENCES

Bessonart, J., *Le Lien et les masques*, Paris, 1983.
Coulon, Madeleine, *La Maternité et les sages-femmes*, Arpin, 1982.
Le Goff, Joelle, *Naître à la maison*, St Georges de Lévéjac, 1981.

INTRODUCTION

FINLAND

Professional training for midwives began in Finland in the mid-eighteenth century. In the nineteenth century it was the first country in the world to base practice on the work of the Hungarian doctor Semmelweiss who demonstrated that the hands of any person attending a woman in childbirth must be scrupulously clean.

Midwives have a central position in the system of care offered to women in childbirth today. Out of thirteen or fourteen antenatal visits, a woman is cared for by midwives exclusively in ten of them. (On the other occasions she is seen by a GP.) There is good follow-up, and a high-risk woman who does not attend a midwives' centre is visited at home by a midwife. Midwives are responsible for all straightforward deliveries.[1]

This chapter examines the background to Finnish midwifery, looks at what is happening to midwives at present, and discusses the inherent conflict between the woman-centred skills of the midwife and an invasive, high-technology obstetrics.

NOTE

1 J.M.L. Phaff (ed.), *Perinatal Health Services in Europe* (World Health Organisation), Croom Helm, 1986.

THE FINNISH MIDWIFE AND HER RENEWED CHALLENGES

LEENA VALVANNE

INTRODUCTION

In terms of perinatal mortality statistics Finland is near the top of the league table. Development during the last five decades has been breathtaking. In 1936, 374 women out of 69,600 who gave birth died in childbirth or from complications during pregnancy, while the perinatal death rate was forty-three per million live births. In 1985 there were four deaths among 62,300 women giving birth and the perinatal death rate was down to 7.3 per 1,000. While one-third of the mothers who gave birth in the 1930s had no qualified assistance, currently all pregnant women go to a hospital for their confinement.

Today childbirth in Finland is centralised, labour is mostly induced, the strength of contractions is regulated, the condition of the foetus is electronically supervised and any deviation from the norm met with technical intervention or medication. Giving birth is regarded as a critical medical situation, as an illness. Even uncomplicated pregnancies receive the same, centralised treatment in specialised wards – just in case.

So much for the mothers. What about the child? From the comfortable, safe darkness of the womb, children are propelled into a brightly lit world where people clatter, shout, and treat them like objects. The child is delivered violently, separated from his mother, left alone, abandoned.

In various parts of the world women are calling for a fundamental change in what has become in the western world a common attitude towards childbirth. These technical methods interfere in the course of the confinement and use force in the treatment of the newborn. Today, in the mid-1980s, this protest movement has reached the Scandinavian countries. Social changes in Finland have necessarily had consequences for the Finnish midwife: her work, her role in society, her tasks in open health care and in hospitals. They have confronted her with new challenges.

THE HISTORY OF MIDWIFERY IN FINLAND

Popular midwifery

Before the first scientifically-trained birth attendants arrived in the seventeenth century, childbirth at tenders were doing their work in smoke saunas, the chimneyless bathhouses of the Finnish provinces. Only these trusted, wise women were competent to conduct childbirth, to control that mysterious happening, and able to feel at home in that tense, magical atmosphere. In popular belief they had a clearly defined place. They knew what was to be done. They knew the prayers, spells and charms to compel the spirits of water and earth. They had their own herbs and concoctions to treat the women in their care.

However, these folk-healers were not very dependable. They could deal with difficulties only with spells or force. The results were predictable; but no very great fuss was made if the child or the mother, or both, were lost in the process.

The beginning of midwifery as a profession

A physician from Stockholm, Johan von Hoorn, trained in obstetrics at the Hôtel Dieu hospital in Paris, and arranged regular training for midwives in Finland. Finland was then under Swedish rule and the Swedish Royal Medical Board granted Hoorn permission to train midwives on six-week courses. In

1697 Hoorn published the first textbook on midwifery. Its vivid and graphic descriptions satisfied the requirements of gynaecology for several decades to come in Sweden and Finland. The midwife's tasks were specified as follows: 'To give good advice to the pregnant, assist the suffering, and after the confinement help the woman in childbed and the newborn.' The midwife's task did not end with delivery.

In 1711 the first regulations for midwives in Sweden and Finland were issued. The midwife had to pass an exam at the Collegium Medicum. Persons without the necessary competence were prohibited from exercising the profession of midwifery under penalty of fines. In 1723 a royal circular letter required county governors to order functionaries in towns and communities to find suitable people to enrol on Hoorn's courses. It evoked no response in Finland.

Regulations for midwives in 1777

When the Institute of Statistics was founded in 1749, the authorities became aware that one-third of children born in Ostrobothnia from 1749 to 1773 and as many as one-half of those born in South-Ostrobothnia died during their first year. Mortality was high among the childbearing women as well. One of the reasons for this was that there were no trained midwives in Finland, able both to assist women in childbirth and to advise them about child rearing. In places where infant mortality was highest, it was found that women neglected to breastfeed their children and had instead been 'horn-feeding' (an early form of bottle-feeding).

Thanks to the efforts of their mayor, the burghers of Pietarsaari set out to find a suitable woman to train as midwife. They sought someone who would be 'god-fearing and conscientious, of good reputation and name, about 40 years of age, patient and compliant, quick to apprehend and reasonably broad-minded. She must not be coarsely built nor fat.' It was thought to be a good thing if she were literate, so as to be able to read books in order to improve her professional skill. In 1751 the good burghers succeeded in finding a person who suited their requirements. Her name was Margareta Forssman and she was sent to Stockholm to train. Presumably the first Finnish midwife, she gradually found some followers and a new regulation for midwives, the first encompassing the whole realm of Sweden and Finland, was issued in 1777. Its aim was to ensure that each parish in the country would have at least one trained midwife. In Finland this seemed to be an unattainable goal. People held that the community was well able to do without a 'midwife mamselle'. There was a shortage of funds and complications ensuing from two different languages being spoken in the country to consider. Nor was the profession of a midwife enviable: the salary was small. Pregnant women continued to turn to their own chosen helpers.

The beginning of midwife training in Finland

The peace treaty between Sweden and Russia in 1809 heralded a new era in Finnish midwifery. The only Institute for midwives' training was in Sweden, now beyond the border of the realm. Contact had become difficult. In 1811 a 'Collegium Medicum', later the National Board of Health, was founded. This Collegium Medicum was allowed to establish a maternity hospital in Turku. The hospital had eight beds; it was intended to serve as a training hospital for midwives. Training lasted from six months to one year and instruction was given in Swedish only.

In 1833 the training of midwives was made the responsibility of the university and moved to Helsinki. The country now had a training institution for midwives; but still in 1857 there were only ninety-seven graduate midwives, and most of these were in towns. In 1859 new regulations for midwives were issued: training was to last two years, and it was to be given in the Finnish language as well as Swedish. The students were required to be able to read and write. Their tasks now included giving vaccinations. However, the situation hardly improved: in 1872 one-third of the country's communities still lacked a midwife.

A new regulation for midwives was issued in 1879. Student midwives were now to be instructed in 'mechanical confinement'. Midwives were to have the right to do forceps deliveries. But the duration of the training was reduced to one year.

In the late 1890s the principal of the training institute, Professor Gustaf Henricius, protested against the short training period and other inadequacies. He submitted numerous motions for their amendment. But it was not until 1920 that his proposed reforms were carried into effect.

The midwife's work and her training during Finland's autonomy

While Finland as the Grand Duchy of Finland was connected with the Russian Empire, instruction for students of midwifery aimed mainly at teaching them how to conduct a confinement competently. Yet the midwife, working among the poor, was constantly confronted with other problems as well. Housing conditions were wretched, sanitation non-existent. It was not easy to work according to course instructions. The midwife had to be resourceful and ingenious when there were no washing facilities and no clothing for mother or child. Moreover the midwife herself was viewed with suspicion in the community with the result that she often earned less than a farmhand or a servant girl.

However, the end of the last and the beginning of the twentieth century proved to be a favourable period for Finnish midwifery. The number of trained midwives quickly grew when instruction began to be given in Finnish in 1859. The first Finnish textbook for students of midwifery, the *Textbook for Finnish Midwives*, appeared in 1861. Now, for the first time, attention was paid to cleanliness. Carefully worded instructions for washing one's hands and the new concern about hygiene brought about a spectacular drop in perinatal mortality.

Towards the end of the nineteenth century communal life in Finland also revived. The more enlightened among the town and community elders at last became aware of the importance of the midwife's work for the health of the population. Maternity hospitals were founded; maternity wards were added to the provincial hospitals. However, at the end of the century 75 per cent of women still gave birth at home without the help of a qualified assistant.

About the same time midwives became aware of their own interests. In 1896 Professor Henricius founded *Kätilölehti* (*The Midwives' Journal*). By means of this journal, Professor Henricius gave postgraduate training to midwives who had already graduated from his institute. He awakened the strong feeling of solidarity that still characterises the profession, the strong endeavour of midwives both to improve their social and economic standing and to raise their professional competence and to make their work more meaningful.

In 1920 the statute 'On Exercising the Profession of a Midwife and on Maternity Hospitals' was published. In the same year an Act was issued 'On the Placing of Midwives in County Communities and on their Salaries'. This was an important step towards improving the standing of midwives; in the communes there had to be at least one midwife for every 5,000 inhabitants.

A new statute in 1937 officially expanded midwifery to encompass all maternity care: care and treatment of women in pregnancy, childbirth and lying-in, and of the newborn.

The 1944 legislation

Overall guidelines for maternity work had been drawn up as early as the 1930s. But it was not until 1944 that Acts were issued on community antenatal clinics, community midwives and local public health nurses. These Acts created a nationwide organisation in Finland with responsibility for maternity care and child health care. The tasks and the standing of the midwife within the framework of this organisation were now firmly established. Admittedly the National Health Act, issued in 1972, repealed these Acts. But the principles of maternity care in Finland were laid down by the Act of 1944.

The National Board of Health supervises maternity care throughout the country. The inspector, a trained midwife, a professor of gynaecology and a group of specialists are in charge of maternity care.

In 1938 a remarkable Act on maternity assistance was issued. A condition for receiving social benefit under this law was that the mother-to-be should avail herself of the services of maternity care before the end of the fourth month of her pregnancy. The frequency of visits to maternity care centres showed a distinct increase as a result of this legislation and the Act of 1944. Moreover the 1944 Act was the death-blow to the corps of self-taught midwives. In 1954 one woman only out of 1,000 gave birth without a qualified assistant. The battle between self-taught and trained midwives had thus lasted 200 years.

But it was not just maternity and child care centres that were built in Finland. In the 1950s and 1960s, a network of central and provincial hospitals was created covering the whole country. This meant that women increasingly went to a maternity ward or a hospital to have their babies instead of staying at home. While 41 per cent of children had been born at home in 1944, and 25 per cent in 1954, this number had plummeted to 3 per cent by 1964, and in 1974 a woman who had not been to hospital for her confinement was the exception that proved the rule. The role of the central hospitals in guiding maternity work was ever more clearly accentuated. This development brought considerable changes in the tasks of midwives employed at the maternity centres. But on the other hand, ever since the 1930s midwives had been trained to respond to the challenges of work in maternity care.

Midwife training

In 1934 the training of midwives was separated from the university, an independent institute being founded for the purpose. The training programme concurrently underwent certain long-planned changes. The course was extended to two years; for a nurse who had already graduated a thirteen-month course in midwifery was scheduled. The training programme was revised as well. The most far-reaching reform was the inclusion of maternity consultation into the curriculum of the school. Furthermore, systematic training in child care was initiated.

The changes effected in the training of midwives in 1940 were fundamental and far-reaching. New subjects were included in the curriculum: gynaecology, care of TB patients, psychoprophylaxis, medical hygiene, community care. Along with theoretical instruction students were now given practical training in obstetric and gynaecological wards, in orphanages and child care centres. Students spent two months at maternity guidance and consultation centres and a further two months in a rural community as assistant to the community midwife.

THE FINNISH MIDWIFE UNDER PRESSURE OF CHANGE

The role of the Finnish midwife is well defined by the words of the specialist commission of the World Health Organisation, in a definition formulated in 1966 as follows:

> She must be able to give necessary supervision, care and advice to women during pregnancy, labour and the postpartum period, to conduct deliveries on her own responsibility and to care for the newborn and the infant. This care includes preventive measures, the detection of abnormal conditions in mother and child, the procurement of medical assistance and the execution of emergency measures in the absence of medical help. The work should also involve antenatal education and preparation for parenthood. It extends to certain areas of gynaecology, family planning and child care.

What, then, is the real meaning of the words, 'supervision, care and advice'? In practice at a maternity centre it has meant checking weight, blood pressure and urine, taking blood samples, checking the size of the womb, and the growth, condition and health of the foetus. And then, of course, advising the mother about nutrition and her general well-being. After the confinement the midwife evaluates the general state of health of mother and child, and on subsequent visits checks whether the woman's body has returned to its normal state. The midwife also helps with family planning. Psychoprophylaxis is considered an essential part of prenatal service.

At a maternity hospital the midwife conducts normal deliveries on her own. She can administer local anaesthetics, perform an episiotomy, stitch the perineum, and give intramuscular injections. On a physician's instructions she can initiate labour and give intravenous injections. In principle the midwife is responsible for mother and child in the maternity ward.

The midwife's role and her tasks both outside and in the hospitals are clearly defined. During pregnancy the doctor has the medical responsibility. The midwife, however, is the person who remains close to the case, observing, giving guidance in health care and social problems, and in psychoprophylaxis.

In the 1960s there was a development which confronted the Finnish midwives with breathtaking changes.

The reform of midwife training in 1968

A statute issued in 1968 discontinued the two years' study course for students of midwifery. From then on they were trained on the basis of a nurse's training only. The period of training was shortened from thirteen months to nine months and the essential out of hospital training in guidance centres and rural communities was abolished. Consequently, the students were trained for hospital work only. This breaking down of the midwife's training was defended with the assertion that midwives were no longer needed outside hospitals, since 'nobody is born at home any more'. The midwife's work was considered to be a narrow specialist field which, in principle, did not differ much from the work of a public health nurse in rural communities, except that the midwife had to take care of the pregnant women in the community.

The rapid transformation of Finland from an agrarian into an industrial society, urbanisation, and the fact that most confinements now took place in maternity hospitals were naturally reflected in the midwife's work. The National Health Act welded the two professions of midwifery and public health nursing into one, the profession of a health worker. At the same time the professional associations of the health workers demanded the abolition of the 'old organisations, and their assimilation into a single strong and influential organisation, a pressure group able to attend to this group's interests'. The Federation of Midwives was on the list of organisations to be abolished. During the 1970s, people used to speak about midwifery as 'the dying profession'.

However midwives tenaciously continued to fight for their training, their status in society and their professional independence; to fight for survival. The battle has not been fought in vain. An Act that came into force in 1987, and the statute that followed, state that midwifery is one of the professions of health work, on an equal footing with the other professions. That is to say, it is a profession that has its own training and final examination (equivalent to the training of a health care worker and the four training courses for nurses). The amended training courses for midwives have already begun. The job description of a graduate midwife contains, in addition to out of hospital and hospital care of her patients, the whole area of gynaecological health care. The training builds on the basic ten years' schooling and takes four and a half years. It provides competence also for jobs which have traditionally been thought to belong to graduate (SRN) nurses.

Nor has the Federation of Finnish Midwives lost its battle to preserve its independence. It still exists as an independent organisation and its membership shows a promising increase. Only the character of the organisation has changed. According to its new statutes it is a professional ideological organisation that has entrusted the protection of its interests to the umbrella organisation of health professionals, Tehyry.

The role of the midwife outside the hospital

Over the years, the Finnish community has changed a great deal. In the 1980s the midwife finds herself facing new challenges. Public values have been greatly modified as have guiding principles, life attitudes, ideals and expectations. The family has changed as well. It is smaller and the status of the child is not what it was.

In the 1950s, when the midwife was no longer attending home births, her first and foremost task was to ensure a safe and healthy pregnancy. There was a shortage of hospital beds; even serious complications had to be treated at home. Women who had moved into the cities from the countryside were often rootless, helpless, and exploited. They lacked that support of the elder generation which their mothers, living in the country among their kin, had still had. It often rested with the midwife to guide these women in the simplest things of daily life: hygiene, care of the newborn, nutrition of the child and herself, and home management. It was factual and tangible help and care.

The standard of living and standard of education improved considerably during the 1960s. Women were an important part of the labour force and children were highly valued. For the midwife the developments of this decade meant that her task changed from actively assisting to guiding, giving advice and offering information. The midwife gave clear-cut instructions without much discussion of her patient's needs and wishes. As before, the emphasis was on assuring the physical well-being of the mother and, increasingly, of the foetus as well.

Technical advances in the 1970s meant that more and more women were sent for ultrasonic or amniotic fluid examinations. Careful screening and the top-class technical equipment of the obstetric wards of the maternity clinics was said to make child-birth easier and safer. But the mother-to-be began to see herself as a patient; her confidence in her health was shaken. A pregnant woman coming for maternity guidance is besieged by many thoughts and cares: fears and hopes on behalf of the child, about parenthood and the changes it would cause, about practical problems concerning job and livelihood, her relations with her husband, and loneliness. Midwives started to question whether their patients really needed so much scientific assistance. The focal point of the guidance given at the maternity centre began to return to emotional values, and guidance became reciprocal interaction between midwife and family. At the turn of the decade new vistas opened for the midwife.

New developments at the hospital

'In the 1960s having a baby was a speeded-up conveyor-belt game,' one of the women whose child had been born in that decade once said, describing her experience at the maternity clinic. Taking childbirth from home to clinic may have improved the physical safety of mother and child, but the mother's feelings during the ordeal were not discussed. The clinic's delivery rooms were big and spacious, accommodating several women. The women were seldom instructed to relax or to breathe in a certain manner, for hospital midwives no longer knew how to prepare a woman for delivery. Women in labour were not allowed to be active. They had to lie on their backs throughout. There was no privacy in the delivery room. People came and went.

And how did the child fare? Bright lights, spot lamps, loud voices, routine workers with briskly grasping hands. No one had taught the hospital midwife what the newborn was trying to convey through her expressions, gestures, and cries.

Nevertheless, the hospital midwife found satisfaction in her work because of her independent status in Finnish hospitals. She was relied upon; she was trusted. But in the 1960s the delivery room was invaded by machines. The midwife's stethoscope, her interpretation of the frequency and strength of the foetal heart sounds, were put aside. Their place was taken by CTG-curves and microblood samples, even if in the beginning heart tocography was only used for risk cases. In the delivery room the midwife's role underwent a change. 'The physician, the technique and the procedures imposed themselves between the midwife and the mother,' as one long-standing midwife put it. But it was not only the delivery room that changed. The nursery in the same unit experienced the same technical invasion. The midwife was assigned the task of always keeping at hand the necessary equipment to revive a newborn in poor condition. The midwife had to be able to provide artificial respiration. She also had to monitor babies at risk after they were born. The midwife was now both the obstetrician's and the paediatrician's right hand. But did that mean she was being transformed into the technical assistant of the physician-technicians?

Development accelerated in the 1970s. CTG-curves began to be compulsory for all pregnant women. 'No birth without machines' might have been the slogan. Birth was actively interfered with, induced, checked, accelerated. The physicians affirmed that there were always clear indications for induction of labour. However, midwives admitted that the manner of confinement depended greatly on the time of day; the midwife's role was different in the evening and at night, when the doctors were not around to give orders about which procedures should be taken. In the 1970s, birth was induced on average in every second woman. Different maternity hospitals had different figures, but two-thirds of women in labour in major hospitals underwent amniocentesis and between 1977 and 1980 were given oxytocics.

Technical development led to the opinion that small maternity hospitals were not safe for parturients, who now had to be brought together in big, well-equipped hospitals. In 1964 Finland had 132 maternity hospitals. In 1980 only fifty were left. At the same time the number of caesareans rose from an average of 4 to 14 per cent. In the biggest hospitals it exceeded 20 per cent.

Did anyone think of the mothers' feelings? Yes. At the same time as midwives were preparing their patients at the maternity guidance centres for a positive experience during labour by teaching them psychoprophylaxis, doctors in maternity hospitals were offering them effective anaesthesia in the form of epidurals, sometimes given as paracervical anaesthesia. The cases receiving epidural anaesthesia varied from 10 per cent to more than 30 per cent. Sometimes the doctors themselves are willing to acknowledge that anaesthetics were too freely used. Something we could call an epidural mentality had arisen.

The pressures to which Finland's midwives were subjected by the Act on national health and the reform of the training of midwives left their mark on the decade of rapid development. While machines occupied the delivery room, one-third of the profession went to the training institutes for nursing the sick for supplementary training, in order not to lose their bread-and-butter jobs. Those who remained were given the more exacting jobs, in the first place in the delivery rooms. In addition to their own jobs, these women now had to bear the responsibility for work performed in the wards, for those patients who had already given birth, as well as in the wards of those who had not, where they now had to supervise and assist personnel lacking the necessary competence. During this decade the maternity hospital midwives worked under great stress. The result was that when the call for innovations came at the beginning of the 1980s, it was rejected by the overworked midwives as well as by the doctors.

The innovation came in the form of three slogans: psychoprophylaxis, birth without violence, and natural birth.

Psychoprophylaxis

In October 1963, Dr Roger Hersilie, senior physician of the Lamaze Hospital, Paris, held a course on 'the psychoprophylactic method to achieve painless birth'. In addition to 100 midwives from the Scandinavian countries, eleven midwives from Finland participated, and they were so enthusiastic about what they had learned that next year the Finnish Federation of Midwives invited Hersilie to lecture in Finland and his method was included in the Institute's teaching course.

One of the important gains of psychoprophylaxis was that for the first time fathers were invited into the delivery room. Here in Finland we really had to do battle about this issue. In the beginning even the midwives were opposed to the idea. They thought men created a disturbance, criticised, were exacting, and spoilt the relation between the mother and her midwife. However, the main opposition came from the doctors. The doors of some hospitals remained firmly closed against the fathers. It was not until in 1981 the booklet *Operation Family* was published, which argued the importance of the father's presence during labour and for future family relations, that the antagonism of the maternity hospitals' senior physicians slowly began to give way. The situation today is that about 60 per cent of fathers participate both in courses and in births; for the first-timers this figure is 80 per cent. In some hospitals the father is allowed to be present even at a caesarean. The hospital midwives' attitude has completely changed. Today they say, 'The child's father is the best pain relief for its mother.'

Birth without violence

In the mid-1970s, Finnish parents who had read about Frédérick Leboyer's methods started to express a wish that their child should have a gentle birth. And by the end of the 1970s, Leboyer's ideas were widely known. In the autumn of 1980 Leboyer himself came to Finland to visit the Gynaecological Clinic of the Central Hospital of Helsinki where he showed films and answered questions. He showed how we receive the child: as if it were a parcel. We measure, weigh, examine, take down notes. And then he showed how we might welcome our children: gently, lovingly, taking in our hands a being endowed with keen perception and feeling, a scared new human being who will bear this moment of his arrival with him during his whole life.

Leboyer also visited the delivery room of the clinic and at some deliveries taking place there he demonstrated how a birth without violence was conducted. 'His artless and unassuming, calm and still powerful personality, his deferential attitude towards life made a profound impression on all of us,' one of those who had been present said later. Leboyer also showed how a caesarean child, too, can be received according to the principles of gentle birth.

After he had gone, discussion of his principles grew. They found both supporters and adversaries. There were various points of view among the midwives. The most convinced supporters were those who had been present at the confinements

Leboyer had conducted. The Finnish translation of Leboyer's book was published to coincide with his visit, and pregnant women began sending lists of their wishes to the chief physicians of maternity hospitals. With a few notable exceptions the doctors reacted scornfully and negatively. One sympathetic physician said,

'In Finland the physicians are above all other things concerned that the child be born healthy and they make use of all achievements of medical science at the delivery, to achieve this purpose. Thus birth becomes a cold, logically built system. At the same time we forget that birth is a psychosocial happening, charged with strong feelings, in the course of which the relationship of the parents towards the child and towards each other is built. Medical science does not mention this, but medical science, practically speaking, never remembers that man is endowed with feelings.'

Gradually Leboyer's principles became known. But today in many hospitals parents themselves must have a clear picture of what it is they want, and very often they also have to make sure that their wishes are complied with. Often, the midwives are likely to stick with the former ingrained routine in their handling of the child: the first meeting of mother and child may be just a fleeting moment, when the mother, let alone the whole family, hardly has time to see or hold her baby.

Natural birth
1979 marked the beginning of the WHO Research and Development Programme, intended to oppose 'the ever stronger tendency to specialisation and technological take-over of the health care system'. It was an endeavour to emphasize human sympathy and an approach that was centred on the human beings involved, on their problems.

There were health centres and hospitals in Finland which embraced these ideas. Since even some maternity guidance centres and maternity hospitals became involved, a number of midwives both outside and in hospitals had to go along with these endeavours. The scope of the midwives' work, both in hospitals and in the guidance centres, expanded, and touched upon deeper problems. Hints on the direction in which development should move in Finland were received from international sources in other ways as well.

In September 1979 the Finnish Federation of Midwives arranged a birth training seminar to which Sheila Kitzinger was invited as lecturer. The seminar attracted 450 participants, midwives working at both guidance centres and hospitals. Sheila Kitzinger's psychosexual emotional approach to birth was new to midwives in Finland. It was a new idea that giving birth could be conceived as the climax of a couple's relationship, a crowning, passionate and creative act. She criticised the western approach to birth, where the woman in labour is strapped to the bed and made to go through parturition in the wholly unnatural supine position. She taught touch relaxation, touch breathing and a natural treatment of the second phase of labour, and stimulated a gradually developing change of attitude in the midwife profession. She awakened interest and also a timid, slowly increasing wish to experiment with something new.

Overseas contacts also improved. A group of Finnish midwives visited Michel Odent's clinic at Pithiviers where they saw for themselves that here birth had been given back to women. Three Finnish participants, one of whom was a midwife, attended the Active Birth Movement's first international conference in London in 1982.

When corresponding conferences were arranged on a national level in, among other countries, Denmark and Norway, the Finnish Federation of Midwives was at last successful in arranging a similar conference in Finland in February 1985. The conference was attended by both obstetricians and paediatricians and also by midwives employed both outside and in hospitals. Although the opportunities to gain insight into the basics of this new approach and the principles of active birth were greatly limited because of the very negative reaction of the physicians who had supervised the arrangement of the conference, the message of the organisers considerably broadened the minds of participants.

During the last few years there has been a lively dialogue between the two antagonistic camps: the supporters of natural and Active Birth methods and those who speak for high technology. The most rigorous adversaries of the new movement are the obstetricians, who dismiss the natural birth movement as a return to the primitive state, which would bring back death as a daily visitor to our maternity hospitals.

What about the midwives? Have they submitted to the role of confinement-technicians, subordinated technical assistants to the physicians? Yes and no. There are midwives who want to continue in the old tradition. (And, of course, there are mothers, as well, who prefer the role of the passive patient.) But there are the other midwives, those influenced by Frédérick Leboyer and Sheila Kitzinger, who have actively begun to gather more information about this new movement and have begun to put the principles into practice. They let the woman in labour move about freely, take a heart curve now and then, and recommend sitting in a rocking chair or a comfortable sack-chair. They have managed to bring crawling mattresses into the delivery room, where father and mother can be together throughout the birth of their child. The midwives in such hospitals say that physicians were initially opposed to such new-fangled ideas. However, the good results achieved have gradually broken their resistance. These midwives also comment that they get more satisfaction out of their work than before.

A similar positive development has taken place in those hospitals where the maternity clinic has participated in the development programme of the WHO. In these clinics the main target is to achieve, along with safety, a method of treatment which is based on the personal needs of the woman involved, which makes giving birth a positive experience for the mother and lays the foundation for the development of a good relationship between mother, child and father. This change in the treatment of the patients of maternity clinics and maternity wards has been a step towards achieving balance between technology and nature.

Changes *are* taking place, but slowly: the hospitals do not offer enough alternatives, having one's baby at home has been made all but impossible, and preparation courses leading to a natural, active birth are still underdeveloped. So women who want to give birth on their own terms have got together. In 1986, together with some midwives and a few physicians they founded the Association for Natural Birth. The members of this

Association think that the most formidable obstacle to a change in confinement practice is rigidity of practice; this attitude is found as often among physicians and midwives as among the patients of maternity clinics themselves. The goal of the Association is to break this rigidity.

At the beginning of the 1980s a Finnish professor of paediatrics claimed that 'within five years, childbirth practice will undergo a total upheaval'. This upheaval has at last begun. It is the greatest challenge before Finnish midwives today.

REFERENCES

Castrén, Olli, *Äitiysneuvolatoiminnan kehityksestä ja tehtävistä maassamme*, Kätilölehti, 1966:1.

Hako, Matti: 'Kansanomainen lääkintötietous', *Suomalaisen kirjallisuuden seuran toimituksia*, vol. 229, 4.osa, Helsinki, 1957.

Hänninen, Sisko-Liisa, *Kätilötyön vaiheita*, Otava, Helsinki, 1965.

Hickl, E.J., Phaff, J.M.L., Sassi, L. and Valvanne, L., *Midwives in Europe*, Report, Co-Ordinated Medical Research, 1974 Programme, Council of Europe, Strasbourg, 1975.

Kitzinger, Sheila, 'Synnytysvalmennusseminaari Turun kesäyliopistossa', Turun yliopiston offsetpaino, 1979.

Kitzinger, Sheila, 'The Birth Revolution: The Rise of the Active Birth Movement in Britain', paper given at the Active Birth Movement conference, London, 1982.

Kulmanen, Marjukka, Lintonen, Kati and Rantanen, Raija-Liisa, 'Vain nainen sen tietää', *Suomalainen synnytys*, WSOY, Porvoo-Helsinki-Juva, 1985.

Leboyer, Frédérick: *Pour une naissance sans violence*, Seuil, 1980.

Lempeä syntymä, Tammi, Helsinki, 1981.

Luonnonmukainen synnytys, *Gummerus*, Jyväskylä-Helsinki, 1985.

Odent, Michel, *Birth Reborn*, Pantheon Books, 1984.

Pitkänen, Heikki, *Äitiyshuoltotyön saavutuksia maassamme*, Kätilölehti, 1960:6.

Reinilä, Anna-Maria, *Pirttimuorit ja paarmuskat*, Kätilölehti, 1965:1.

Sorvettula, Maija, *WHO:n hoitotyön ohjelma ja sen toteuttaminen*, Kätilölehti, 1983:2.

SVT, *Väestöosa I*, 1985.

Toivanen, Hilkka, *Vanhemmaksi kasvamisen tukeminen äitiyshuollossa*, Kätilölehti, 1983:2.

Valvanne, Leena, *Kansanomaisesta synnytysavusta tämän päivän äitiyshuoltoon*, Kätilölehti, 1966:10

Valvanne, Leena, *Keinutuoli synnytyshuoneessa eli miten kätilötötä on kehitetty ja syvennetty Kanta-Hämeen keskussairaalassa*, Kätilölehti, 1983:2.

Valvanne, Leena, *Luonnonmukaisuus ja inhimillisyys lapsen syntyessä*, Kätilölehti, 1986:2.

Valvanne, Leena, *Rakkautta pyytämättä, Valtakunnankätilö muistelee*, Tammi, Helsinki, 1986.

Valvanne, Leena, *Teknologian vaikutus synnytyksen hoidon luonteeseen*, Kätilölehti, 1972:12.

Wagner, Marsden, *Lapsen saanti Euroopassa*, Kätilölehti, 1985:2.

WHO, Europe, *Having a Baby in Europe*, Report on a study, Denmark, 1985.

INTRODUCTION

THE NETHERLANDS

In the Netherlands birth is considered a normal physiological process. Care is, on the whole, non-interventionist. Women walk around during labour, intravenous fluids are not generally given, attendants wear no masks and gowns, sterile drapes are not used, other family members are present, and episiotomies are performed in only about 8 per cent of all deliveries.

Midwives are independent practitioners responsible for the regulation of their own profession. This has been the case since as long ago as 1885. Reimbursement of their fees is made through the state health insurance system. Until recently, insurance did not pay for a low-risk woman to go into hospital to have her baby, and 96 per cent of all midwife-assisted births took place at home. Nowadays the economic incentive for home birth has been reduced because indications for hospital birth have been extended and insurance companies readily cover the cost. Still, however, 'home delivery does not have the stigma it has in other countries – that of anti-social behaviour by a self-neglecting subculture.' (Joop Offerman, 'The Netherlands', *Childbirth Education*, Fall, 1985, pp. 26–31).

Eighty per cent of midwives are direct-entry and only 20 per cent are nurse-midwives. Two out of every five babies are born with midwife care alone, without a doctor being called. The perinatal mortality for these midwife-assisted births is the lowest in the world, approximately two per 1,000.

Throughout the Netherlands rates of induction and of caesarean section are very low compared with other European countries, and anaesthesia is rarely used. Perinatal mortality comes second only to Sweden and Finland, and is much below most other industrialised countries, including the United States.

The Netherlands are unique in that a midwife conducting a home birth can be assisted by a trained home help maternity nurse who gives practical postpartum care as long as the woman needs it, including looking after any other children, and this care is also reimbursed by insurance.

In the following chapter two practising midwives, Beatrijs Smulders and Astrid Limburg, discuss the background and present politics of midwifery in the Netherlands and talk about the challenges it is facing.

OBSTETRICS AND MIDWIFERY IN THE NETHERLANDS

BEATRIJS SMULDERS AND ASTRID LIMBURG

INTRODUCTION

The midwife in Dutch society assumes a unique and interesting role in the context of medical practice. People often wonder why the position of midwives, and the nature of obstetric care in the Netherlands, differs from those in other western countries. The answer lies chiefly in its obstetric and social history. The interaction of certain medical developments and social trends has produced the current system in the Netherlands where the Dutch midwife operates independently.

Dutch midwives are engaged in a continuous effort to facilitate what may be described as a 'natural' birth process, with medical intervention reserved only for emergencies. Nowadays, however, doctors, armed with new high-tech medical systems available only in hospital settings, are denouncing the independent midwife. Dutch midwives, for their part, have taken a firm stand against the medicalisation of childbirth.

THE EARLY HISTORY OF MIDWIFERY IN HOLLAND

In most countries, the right to perform obstetrics independently, without supervision, is reserved for licensed doctors. Holland is an exception. A Dutch midwife can legally practice obstetrics without the supervision of a doctor when pregnancies and deliveries show no indication of medical complications.

In the seventeenth century, for example, nearly all deliveries were performed by midwives. Obstetric surgeons would be called in to assist in deliveries only in the event that some surgical procedure was deemed necessary by the midwife. During the last 300 years, the Dutch midwife's control over obstetrics has gradually lessened into more of a sharing role with the licensed obstetricians. By 1965, only 35 per cent of deliveries were performed by midwives. Recently, however, there has been a trend to return to 'natural' childbirth. By 1984, the percentage of midwife-assisted deliveries had increased to 43 per cent.

The history of midwifery in the Netherlands is fascinating. In the sixteenth century, there were three groups of individuals involved in birthing: the '*doctores medicinae*', academics who studied obstetrics in universities but tended to shy away from actual deliveries; obstetric surgeons, who provided assistance when complications occurred; and midwives, who assumed the vast majority of the work. The surgeons were carrying out such procedures as caesarean sections; female surgeons did not exist.

Interestingly, during the seventeenth and eighteenth centuries a minor battle of the sexes occurred in Dutch midwifery. While the practice of midwifery was, and continues to be, a primarily female occupation, male midwives entered the scene and challenged their female counterparts. Many of the male 'midwives' were actually obstetric surgeons who wanted to expand their business beyond formal surgical procedures. Even then the surgeons could use certain new technologies, as basic as the use of forceps, in deliveries, whereas traditional female midwives maintained 'natural' childbirths without tools.

The development of forceps presents an interesting case of application, or often misapplication, of technology. In many instances, forceps could be used effectively with difficult deliveries. On the other hand, improper use of forceps could lead to brain damage or other impairments in the infant, and laceration of the mother.

The male surgeon acting as midwife nonetheless became popular among the wealthier classes in Holland. In 1784, Terne described the practice of obstetrics as inadequate, with excessive mortality and injury to mother and child. He attributed this to the increase in deliveries by surgeons who were not properly trained. At that time, surgeons did not have to attend universities. The competition between surgeons and midwives spread throughout Europe, as attested to by the French midwife and writer Louisa Bourgeois in 1626.

Female midwives, however, gradually gained the respect of the Dutch surgeons. The Dutch midwives did most of the work and were provided with more assistance in the form of training from the medical establishment. Books by Louisa Bourgeois and the famous German midwife Justine Sigemundin were quickly translated by Dutch surgeons for the benefit of Dutch midwives. Obstetric surgeons who espoused the role of midwives included Cornelis van Solingen (1641–87), Hendrik van Deventer (1651–1724), and Petrus Camper (1722–89). The English doctor Smellie, on the other hand, criticised midwives, apparently feeling that the female sex had limited competence in medical matters.

In most European countries, female midwives not only faced greater competition from the surgical obstetricians but they were also not allowed entrance into medical education programmes. The influence of the Inquisition, which in part sought to push women back into more traditional, less professional roles, was greater in other parts of Europe than in Holland, the first country in which freedom of religion prevailed. New ideas were tolerated in the Netherlands. The result was that the three groups involved in birthing (academics, the obstetric surgeons, and the midwives) cooperated with one another, rather than jockeying for the dominant position.

The diary of Catherine Schraders, a Dutch midwife whose practice extended for a period of about fifty-two years during the early eighteenth century, reveals that her techniques and procedures were highly professional, even by today's standards (the mortality rate of the mothers delivering was the same as that in the United States in 1936!).

THE NINETEENTH AND EARLY TWENTIETH CENTURIES

The roles of the academic doctors and obstetric surgeons changed in the nineteenth century, and began to infringe more on the territory of the Dutch midwives. The academics began to practise surgery and obstetrics, and the surgeons advanced into internal medicine. In 1865, the politician Thorbecke designed a new law for health policy that sought to define more clearly the roles of these three groups and bring some order to the nation's health programmes.

Thorbecke's law can be summarised as follows. Firstly, all doctors (including surgeons) would have an academic education, part of which would include training in obstetrics. Secondly, midwives were granted an official status, with established authority for making decisions. The midwife was confined, however, to 'normal' deliveries. The rates charged by doctors were also regulated at a higher level, which meant that the midwives were essentially guaranteed sufficient clientele. Thus the midwife became the obstetrician for the poor.

In 1861, the first academy for midwives was founded in Amsterdam. In 1882, a second academy was established in Rotterdam, and a third in 1913 in Heerlen. These schools, which continue to operate today, provided midwives with a solid education and a government-endorsed examination, which had the effect of raising the quality of midwifery in the Netherlands. In 1912 two prominent doctors, Professor De Snoo and Catherina van Tussenbroek, advocated the cause of the Dutch midwife and, as a result, the government extended the education of midwives from two to three years, and incorporated prenatal care. It was also decided that the midwifery academy would remain separate from nursing schools.

THE ESTABLISHMENT OF ORGANISED MATERNITY AID

The institution of maternity aid was first established at a local level in Holland. Maternity aid nurses were trained to take care of mother and child in the first ten days after the delivery. In 1925, the national government endorsed this practice, and the National Institute of Maternity Aid was founded. This development substantially improved the position of Dutch midwives because it relieved them of the post-delivery nursing activities. During the delivery itself, the trained maternity aid nurses would assist the midwives and then assume responsibility for the ten-day post-delivery period. This allowed the Dutch midwife to focus more fully on her medical duties.

When the midwives' share of the obstetric market declined from 59 per cent in 1909 to 48 per cent in 1940, it was primarily due to greater competition from general practitioner doctors. The government once again took measures to protect midwives. In 1941 it was decreed that women covered by national health insurance could not receive reimbursement for fees charged by general practitioners for deliveries if a midwife was established and practising in the vicinity. This law is still in force today, although it has been the subject of controversy for the past several decades. The government, however, stands firm in preserving the institution of midwifery. Further, in 1962 the midwife's fees were increased by 50 per cent.

During this century, the science of obstetrics has continued to develop. Progress in prenatal care has been of great importance, detecting and preventing defects before delivery. Dutch midwives followed these advances closely and their scope of responsibility expanded to incorporate these new sciences. In 1951 the government decreed that the midwife would care for the mother throughout her pregnancy. For example, with external manipulations, the midwife can correct malpositions of the foetus. Midwives also take blood from pregnant women for further examination at clinics. They provide dietary advice; take cervical swabs; use certain medicines during delivery; perform episiotomies when necessary and stitch episiotomies, vaginal tears and perineal ruptures.

THE MIDWIFE IS NO NURSE

Midwives and nurses are trained in different schools in Holland. The Dutch believe that these two professions require totally different attitudes as well as different skills. A nurse has to work within the hierarchy of the hospital, under the supervision of doctors. A midwife, on the other hand, has equivalent rights in the field of obstetrics as general practitioners and she is expected to work independently in the field.

In 1963, the Medical Superintendent published a report on the status of midwives that stated that, as a sign of progress, an increasing number of GPs were moving into obstetrics. The report suggested that it was no longer necessary to protect midwives by laws since with the expansion of the social security system the public could afford obstetric care from doctors. There was also a greater number of GPs working in Holland to provide obstetric care. The report concluded that the national health insurance regulations supporting midwives should be terminated, even though it acknowledged that midwives would still be necessary for an interim transition period. The Medical Superintendent also recommended that a nursing degree be a prerequisite for entering the midwifery academies. He argued that midwives could thereby have some sort of income as post-delivery nurses and work within hospitals or obstetric clinics assisting doctors. Also, they would come in handy whenever a GP was called away from a delivery for an emergency-case.

Clearly, if these recommendations had been adopted by the government the independent midwife and the concept of home delivery would now be relics of the past. Fortunately, however, subsequent government reports took a very different tone and supported the midwife. The Central Committee of Public Health decreed in the 1970s that midwives should have the primary responsibility for normal deliveries, and that GPs would handle non-delivery medical issues.

In Holland the midwife has assumed this unique position in public health because throughout history she has always been able to rely on the support of influential doctors and obstetric surgeons. Midwives received this support at crucial moments, and they won better training and remuneration to improve the overall quality of obstetric care. It is also clear that midwives have represented a more affordable delivery option for the poorer people in Holland. Finally, the government has consistently protected the midwife by guaranteeing her an income, by institutionalising home delivery, and by fully subsidising the maternity aid system. Even now, in the 1980s, midwives are receiving support publicly from prominent professors of obstetrics, support that is finding its way into the policy-making bodies of government. Dutch midwives also formed a professional association in the early twentieth century which continues to advocate the midwives' cause and to provide public education on obstetric care.

THE MIDWIFE AND THE TRADITION OF NATURAL BIRTH

Since midwives have denounced using medical tools, it was in their own interest to keep birth as 'natural' as possible. As long as the birth was kept natural, there would be no need to call in the GP or the obstetrician. As a small entrepreneur, the independent midwife protected her territory, as long as it was not to the detriment of the child or mother. Like all entrepreneurs, the midwife has traditionally relied on word of mouth recommendations to bring her new clients. Today, as in the past, it is in the midwife's interest to perform tasks as efficiently and reliably as possible.

With experience and zeal as her only tools, the midwife has dedicated herself to developing a specific knowledge of the physiology of pregnancy and birth. Her methods are often described as the 'psychosocial' approach to obstetrics, in contrast to the 'medical' approach. These two extremes, the psychosocial and the medical, have a fundamentally different vision of the pregnant woman. In the medical approach, the woman is perceived as a patient, as someone who has a disease and requires treatment, whereas in the midwife's approach, she is considered a healthy person who, with assistance, will achieve something very special.

Nevertheless, in the 1970s the doctor's power and status rose considerably because of many new technological acquisitions. Medicine was increasingly respected. Between 1970 and 1979 the number of midwives remained stable, but there was a sharp increase in the number of gynaecologists – no less than 42 per cent. In the same period the total number of hospitalised births rose from 20 per cent in 1970 to a staggering 46 per cent in 1979. In short, the number of both births and home deliveries fell sharply, whereas the number of hospital deliveries increased. This rise can partly be explained by an increase of so-called voluntary preference to deliver in hospital. For the most part, however, it was due to increasing intervention by obstetricians.

Is hospitalisation warranted? Since every woman is extremely sensitive and vulnerable when the safety of her new baby is at stake, the mother can easily be manipulated by arguments favouring hospitalisation, even if the need for medical attention is

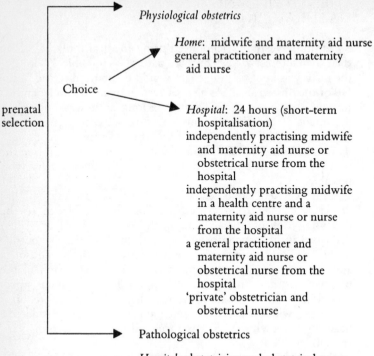

Physiological obstetrics

Home: midwife and maternity aid nurse
general practitioner and maternity
    aid nurse

Hospital: 24 hours (short-term
    hospitalisation)
independently practising midwife
    and maternity aid nurse or
    obstetrical nurse from the
    hospital
independently practising midwife
    in a health centre and a
    maternity aid nurse or nurse
    from the hospital
a general practitioner and
    maternity aid nurse or
    obstetrical nurse from the
    hospital
'private' obstetrician and
    obstetrical nurse

Choice

prenatal
selection

Pathological obstetrics

Hospital: obstetrician and obstetrical nurse
(paediatrician)

not justified. Hospitals also have an incentive to fill their beds, and it is a fact that home deliveries are considerably less costly than those in hospitals.

Data show that in 1979, one out of every three women who was sent to hospital due to an 'expected' medical complication turned out to have an uncomplicated birth. And even though more women seem to be using hospitals for their deliveries, it is clear that giving birth has become less, not more dangerous. We now have the answers to mechanical problems of birth and have solved the problems of hygiene, that can lead to infection and death, which were so prevalent in the nineteenth century. The new problem which has arisen today is the neglect of psychological and emotional aspects of the birth process that has come with medicalisation.

THE MIDWIFE OF TODAY

Two separate teams operate in the field of obstetrics: the obstetrician and the obstetrical nurse take care of pathological obstetrics in the hospital, while the healthy and uncomplicated pregnancies and births are conducted under the guidance of a midwife and a maternity aid nurse at home or in the hospital.

In general one could say that there are two different types of midwife. There is the independently practising midwife who runs her own practice in the city or in the country (in 1986 70.3 per cent of all midwives were independent). And there is the midwife who works in the physiological obstetric unit of a hospital (17.2 per cent in 1986). She performs the physiological prenatal and natal care. In case of pathology she hands over to the obstetrician and assists him. Statistics show that in 1983 the number of hospital-affiliated midwives decreased as compared to the number of independent midwives focusing on home delivery. In 1986 there was a total of 949 midwives, 695 of whom practised independently.

The midwife has traditionally worked alone in her practice. In 1971, 91 per cent of independent midwives practised alone. However, in the last ten years, more midwives have established group practices. In 1981, 28 per cent of all practices consisted of more than one midwife, where the members could share workloads and take holidays more easily. These group practices typically have one midwife providing consultations to pregnant women while another stays 'on-call' to carry out deliveries. Roles are switched on a weekly basis. During the prenatal consultations, the bond of trust established between expectant mothers and midwives is an important element in a successful delivery.

PRENATAL CARE

During her pregnancy the pregnant woman visits the midwife twelve or fourteen times. The midwife takes care of the mother both technically and psychosocially. It is the midwife's task to recognise abnormalities as early as possible. All women with an increased risk factor are screened out and sent to an obstetrician, where many are given what is called a 'medical indication' which warrants hospitalisation for the delivery. Another aspect of the midwife's care is psychological. As pregnant women have become more aware of their needs and demands, more emphasis has been placed on such guidance. The pregnant woman is encouraged to actively and consciously experience the birth process. Although pain is almost inevitable, the mother's fear can be addressed so that she can still enjoy and remember the birth as a meaningful, rich experience. The midwife strengthens the mother's confidence. Fathers are also actively involved in the birth process.

HOME DELIVERY

When a woman gives birth at home, the midwife and the maternity aid nurse are like guests, adapting themselves to the particular circumstances and trying to increase the self-confidence and autonomy of the woman giving birth. Self-confidence is crucial because fear, anxiety and pain form a vicious circle. When a woman experiences giving birth as a natural, creative event, she delivers with more pleasure and with fewer problems. The midwife coaches the woman through the birth process and will always try to avoid any event that might disturb her. For a woman in labour who is disturbed runs the risk of not being able to complete the delivery on her own. All medical intervention, such as the use of forceps or a vacuum extractor, carries a certain risk for mother and child. So there is a clear correlation between a pleasant and a safe delivery. For a safe home birth the presence of a maternity aid nurse to assist the midwife is essential.

THE POSTNATAL PERIOD

The midwife visits the new mother four or five times after the birth. The maternity aid nurse takes extensive notes on all events during the post partum period and problems are discussed with the midwife and the parents. The midwife will seek a solution within the family setting and will always try to prevent the separation of mother and child.

THE LAST CHECK-UP SIX WEEKS POSTPARTUM

The final check-up always takes place in the practice and is done by the midwife who has conducted this particular delivery. Often the mother is accompanied by her partner and the baby. Vaginal examination, haemoglobin level, blood pressure and weight are checked. The midwife does not medically examine the infant, however, since this is done in the Infant Welfare Centre. This visit also has an important psychosocial aspect, since the midwife and the parents discuss the birth experience, their feelings, and also specific issues such as sex and birth control.

THE MIDWIFE AS INSTRUCTOR

In a growing number of hospital and academic clinics, midwives have been incorporated as part of the medical staff. Midwives and obstetricians jointly teach medical students. Medical students are also given the opportunity to attend home deliveries under the supervision of an independent midwife, and to participate in postnatal procedures, if the parents-to-be give permission. Thus, medical students can witness the entire process, one that can be most interesting because the approach is primarily non-interventionist. Future gynaecologists, paediatricians and GPs thereby gain insight into and respect for the midwifery profession, tutored in a sense by the parents who have chosen a natural home birth for their child.

THE CURRENT POSITION OF MIDWIVES IN THE NETHERLANDS

The percentage of midwife-assisted births has remained fairly constant over the last twenty years, and is presently about 43 per cent. The percentage for gynaecologists increased substantially during that period at the expense of deliveries performed by GPs.

The tradition of the independent midwife has contributed to the belief in Holland that delivery is a natural event, and that medical treatment should only be resorted to when there are complications. A balance between gynaecologists and midwives now exists, with neither party holding a monopoly in obstetrics. Many women in Holland have a rich, meaningful and safe experience delivering babies at home. The influence of the home deliverers in our society has been strong, and hospitals have had to adapt their approach to pregnant women.

An obstetric system where all deliveries take place in a hospital is detrimental to both midwives and mothers. The former are degraded to mere obstetrician's aides, losing their independence. The mother is treated as a patient, and is subject to a greater level of medical intervention. In Holland, however, obstetricians have been influenced to meet the particular wishes of women in labour, since it is in their own interest to do so in order to maintain their market share of work. The result is that the doctor's approach to delivering babies in Holland is less interventionist than in other countries. Holland has a low percentage of operative deliveries (10 per cent). In other countries, such as Germany, the United States, Canada, and England, that percentage is much higher (40 per cent). Also, in Holland, the use of anaesthetics is rare during births, and in general, an effort is made in hospitals to create a home-like atmosphere in special birthing rooms.

THE CONFLICT WITH OBSTETRICIANS

A number of Dutch obstetricians support the developments in midwifery. Not surprisingly, others feel that all deliveries should occur in hospital. They argue that every delivery entails risk, and as a result, deliveries should be closely monitored with 'high-tech' equipment. These obstetricians justify their interventionist methods by referring to the decrease of perinatal mortality, which has indeed dropped in the western world. Midwives, however, attribute this development to better public health practices in general and to improved prenatal care. Most women still have a normal pregnancy and delivery. The most frequent complication during the birth process is that the expulsion of the infant is hindered, a problem that is remedied by the application of vacuum extraction or forceps. In reality, only a small percentage of deliveries can truly benefit from 'high-tech' solutions.

The arguments of interventionist doctors can sometimes be misleading when biased interpretations of data are used to scare women into going to hospitals. These obstetricians repeatedly attack the position of midwives and the benefits of home delivery. Their most effective weapon is to tell women in prenatal check-ups that a 'medical indication' may be in order, the costs of which would be covered by national health insurance. The issue of medical indication has both professional and economic consequences. When an obstetrician defines a woman as a medium-risk patient, the obstetrician benefits financially. Every time a woman is referred back to a midwife, the obstetrician loses revenue. The increase in medical indications not only infringes on the working terrain of midwives but also directly affects their income.

The midwife has a powerful and, we feel, legitimate weapon in this modern-day medical conflict. Firstly, there are the genuine benefits of natural birth, both for the mother and for the child. Secondly, the midwife may choose from a number of obstetricians in the area, and can therefore send the pregnant woman to sympathetic doctors.

Who can really determine what is 'normal' or 'abnormal', and when interventions are genuinely appropriate? Midwives and physicians obviously apply different interpretations. The percentage of medical indications rose from 26 per cent in 1971 to 46 per cent in 1979, a period when we know that public health generally continued to improve. In an effort to halt this development, the Medical Board of Advisors to National Health Insurance has recently produced a new list of guidelines regarding medical indications in pregnancy. The objectives of this effort are to forestall the arbitrary issue of medical indications and, indirectly, to clarify the relationship between obstetricians and midwives. Further, it aims to reduce medical costs. Not surprisingly, a number of obstetricians have complained loudly about these guidelines, because their flexibility and, ultimately, revenue base, is restricted. Feelings are running high!

The role of the general practitioner in this conflict is unclear. However, physicians more readily refer their patients to obstetricians because of the medical biases in their own training. Until 1978, the number of home deliveries had been declining every year. Since then more women have chosen to deliver at home.

Since 1978 worried midwives, women's rights groups and consumer organisations have informed pregnant women about the value of the Dutch obstetric system and of the freedom and support to choose different birth alternatives. Conferences have been held, articles have been published, natural birth books have become bestsellers, and television and radio stations have covered the subject extensively. Pregnant women have been made aware of the dangers of unnecessary medical interventions, and the relationship between a 'pleasant' and a 'safe' delivery has been made clear. The information was geared to increase a woman's trust in her own capabilities, and the midwife was always presented as the person who allows women to participate and control their births as actively as possible. Midwives have presented themselves as specialists in normal, pleasant and safe birth.

The result of this publicity and hard work is that home delivery is gaining in popularity in Holland. The midwife is once again respected in Dutch society and midwifery schools are flooded with applications. Midwives participate in the registration of births and other scientific data gathering. Recent research on these obstetric results has also contributed to the midwife's improved status. While the midwife's financial status still trails behind her professional status, the government is currently debating measures to improve that as well.

THE FUTURE

The concept of home delivery and that of the independent midwife have essentially become a single force in Dutch society. If one falters, so does the other. Thus, in trying to improve its position in obstetrics, the midwife community has sought to educate society on the genuine advantages of home delivery. To be effective in this effort, the midwives have realised the need for better organisation, better renumeration, and better public communication on their own part. To reveal the 'facts' about delivery, midwives have also participated more keenly in scientific research. Midwives are taking steps as a group to ensure and improve the quality of their practice. They also face the continuing task of preserving a reasonable dialogue within the medical community, especially with the obstetricians, for the most important aim of Dutch midwives for the future is that all physiological obstetrics should be conducted by midwives and all pathological obstetrics by gynaecologists. The list of medical indications, recently composed, is an important step in the realisation of this indispensable allocation of tasks. Without this allocation of tasks within the organisation of obstetrics total medicalisation is inevitable.

The future of midwives in Dutch obstetrics can be viewed with optimism. However, as demonstrated by events throughout history, the position of the midwife will always be under challenge, particularly in this age of technology. The midwife will have to fight to protect the integrity of an event as natural as pregnancy and birth from the alienating effects of technocratic society. Her best weapons will continue to be education, alertness, creativity, and sensitivity.

At the current time Dutch midwives function as role models for all midwives in the western world. Therefore they feel the extra responsibility to safeguard the facilities that have been built up to provide expectant mothers with a maximum of freedom and yet a high degree of security.

REFERENCES

K. Caranza, *Midwives Caught in the Forceps*, Amsterdam, 1983.

A. Crebas, *The Position of the Independent Midwife in the Netherlands*, Amsterdam, 1986.

R. van Daalen, *Having a Baby in the Netherlands*, Amsterdam, 1986.

S. Gijsel, *The Position of the Dutch Midwife*, Amsterdam, 1984.

E. de Haan and J. Spanjer, *Delivering Better*, Amsterdam, 1985.

G.J. Kloosterman, *The Dutch Journal of Obstetrics*, no 32, 1978, Giving Birth under Supervision: the Coup of the Specialists.

NIVEL, *Registratie Verloskundige Peiling*, 1986.

B. Smulders and A. Crebas, *Task Definition within Obstetric Care in Holland*, Amsterdam, 1987.

B. Smulders and A. Limburg, *Medicalisation and the Home Birth System in Dutch Culture: A Controversy?*, Amsterdam, 1987.

INTRODUCTION

THE MIDWIFE'S ROLE IN MODERN HEALTH CARE

A nurse with midwifery training who then chose to specialise in another area of nursing, once told me that she hated midwifery because 'it's nothing but blood, bottoms, boobs and bedpans'.

In this final chapter, a senior midwife who has experience of working in North America as well as in Britain, and of both home and hospital births, offers a very different view and explores what midwifery is all about. What does it mean to choose midwifery as a vocation? And why should anyone want to assist at the emergence of new life? How is it that some women actually enjoy being midwives?

THE MIDWIFE'S ROLE IN MODERN HEALTH CARE

LESLEY PAGE

Pregnancy and birth occur in a social context, and everyone involved experiences or defines the event differently. For mother, father, family, friends and physician the event has a different meaning.

The first-time mother, for example, may be concerned about her change of status, her changing relationship with her partner and her direct experience of pregnancy. We can imagine her telling her family that she is going to have a baby, and waiting to hear their reaction; we can imagine her mixed feelings, the sickness of early pregnancy, the dreams and happiness and possibly anxiety which she will experience. This is a momentous event for her, one of transformation; it is unique. Of course she wants to keep her baby safe, but this is a minimum, basic need, and she is also concerned with the emotional and spiritual aspects of life. For the mother pregnancy and childbirth mean a major change: life will never be the same again.

Through the eyes of the obstetrician, however, birth is a commonly occurring event, seen many times each day. Birth is defined mainly by its physical attributes. The obstetrician is knowledgeable about and sensitive to medical problems and physical indicators of health. Pregnancy and birth are described in terms of ultrasound, alfa-feto protein levels, and so on. The definition of birth in obstetrical terms is medical.

Midwifery also has its own unique perspective, its own definition of birth. This definition bridges the two perspectives outlined above, and includes both family and physical changes. The unique perspective and approach of midwifery provides the potential of bringing together the two definitions of birth, to provide balance in the health care system, because the tradition of midwifery brings a sensitivity to the spiritual and experiential aspects of birth.

However, present-day midwifery in the industrialised world does not fulfil this role. Where midwives were once the only practitioners in birth, and cared for the family throughout labour and birth and afterwards, the role of the midwife in many health care systems has now become fragmented, and midwives have lost their once powerful position in the lying-in chamber. Today the woman and her family are looked after by different people at different points. This fragmentation of care is in part the result of a more technical age, the many health care professionals involved in care, and the development of hospital-based care.

Today things are changing. People are becoming a little more sceptical about the wisdom and accuracy of technology, and are searching for human and spiritual values in their lives. Similarly, in childbirth we are noticing amongst both families and health care professionals a return to a focus on physiological childbirth, in which the emotional and the spiritual aspects are honoured.

The evidence of this change is seen in the many 'birth movements' which have developed around the world and have been described in this book; natural childbirth, the active birth movement, the maternal health societies, and the many midwives' groups provide some examples.

People are asking for change in the way pregnancy and birth are treated within the health care system, and we need a mediator to bring together the two points of view, and to provide balanced care. Because of the particular characteristics of midwifery, this is the natural role of the midwife.

I am advocating that the role of midwifery is to negotiate a definition of birth which includes both the medical and the family perspectives. In negotiating the two definitions the midwife brings a unique perspective on birth and different approaches to care. These perspectives and approaches are an amalgamation of the traditions of midwifery and the best of scientific perinatal care.

The following five principles derive from the unique perspective of midwifery and should be characteristic of modern midwifery care.

(1) Continuity of care
(2) Respect for the normal
(3) Enabling informed choices
(4) Recognition of birth as more than a medical event
(5) Family-centred care

(1) CONTINUITY OF CARE

I would go so far as to say that midwifery is not midwifery without a basis of continuity of care. Fragmented care is one of the major problems facing childbearing women today. The provision of continuity of midwifery care would be a major step in overcoming the fragmentation which characterises current maternity care.

In the same way as physicians, midwives may choose to provide continuity of care by the organisation of small teams of partnerships. These teams could include student midwives. The team approach often integrates physicians and midwives working together as colleagues, each with their own unique contribution to make to the care of families.

Any change to create a system of care where continuity is possible would require retraining and considerable reorganisation, but would have many advantages. Foremost is the advantage to the mother of knowing her midwives, which is a crucial factor as labour approaches. A very special bond often develops between the mother and family and their midwife, so the time of birth becomes a shared event, celebrated by the family and midwife or midwives alike. Furthermore, the parents will have developed a relationship in which they know they can trust the midwife, and will have had the opportunity to discuss their respective points of view. Knowing the family puts the midwife in an ideal situation to encourage and reassure the parents through labour and birth.

A second advantage is that of safety. Having cared for the woman throughout her pregnancy, the midwife is aware of the health of mother and baby, and their amount of potential reserves for coping with labour. She knows the family's physical and emotional strengths, and knowing at first hand the history of the pregnancy she is able to make more accurate clinical judgments about the course and appropriate management of labour and birth. Then, no less important, she is able to assess the kind of support and teaching the family will need in the postpartum period.

But perhaps the most compelling reason for continuity of care is that it sets the foundation for accountability. It is as important to a midwife as it is to a physician to provide care for the mother in pregnancy, birth and the postpartum, as this enables the midwife to be accountable for care to her families. This accountability to families is an important factor in developing professional autonomy for midwifery.

Postpartum care requires special emphasis, for it has become the Cinderella of perinatal care, yet an aware midwife understands the importance of this time, because it is the period when, after the excitement of the birth is over, the parents need to take the baby into their hearts and lives. This is a time of massive readjustment, and the midwife may play a crucial role in assisting the mother to feed the baby adequately, and in helping the mother and father adjust to parenthood.

(2) RESPECT FOR THE NORMAL

In most parts of the world the midwife is the specialist in normal pregnancy and birth. Her approach is one of confidence in and respect for physiological processes. This is in contrast to an attitude which looks for, and often invites, crisis. The understanding of the finely attuned processes of physiological pregnancy and labour and birth leads to an awareness of the danger of unnecessary intervention, and the cascade of effects which follow. This does not mean, however, that midwives should allow nature to take its course. The modern midwife must be able to diagnose abnormalities. If these occur, she must be able to manage the complication or make the appropriate medical referral.

Avoidance of intervention

The traditional approach of midwifery is to intervene only when absolutely necessary. I believe this includes the use of analgesia and anaesthesia in labour. In an age where we seem to believe we can always improve on nature, where health care is dominated by dramatic technology, and where defensive attitudes on medico-legal issues predominate, it will be a daunting task to re-establish this principle. In Britain, Wendy Savage's case has illustrated the crucial dilemma of our times. We can never provide absolute safety – a small number of babies will always die in birth – but it seems that we are more likely to be exonerated if we have used some form of technical intervention, than if we have not.*

Traditionally, effective midwifery care has been based on a strong foundation of prevention, and so I am faced with the problem of describing an approach to care which is based on common sense judgments and the experience gained in prenatal care. The effects of preventative approaches on outcomes would be a fertile ground for midwifery-based evaluation. In the meantime, I believe we should continue using preventative approaches but, as with everything, with a sense of moderation, and being aware of the potential dangers of any kind of interference.

Another aspect of prevention is often overlooked; if we look at pregnancy outcomes throughout the world we see that the curse of poverty is one of the most important risks to pregnancy and birth. Mortality and morbidity rates are far higher when the family is socially disadvantaged. Hence the major form of prevention may be the provision of adequate food, shelter, and income for disadvantaged groups. Midwives, if adhering to a principle of prevention, need to be involved in the development of social policy, and in the provision of prenatal outreach programmes for particular groups.

* In 1986 Wendy Savage, a consultant obstetrician in London, was suspended from work on the grounds of possible negligence in five cases. After an investigation a year later and a tribunal examination, she was exonerated. In only one of the five cases did the parents make a complaint against her; patients' records were scoured for possible evidence after allegations had been made by her medical colleagues. She works in the community so that pregnant women can avoid the long journey to the hospital antenatal clinic for their check-ups, supports home births, is reluctant to perform unnecessary caesarean sections, and is an advocate of women's rights in childbirth.

The role of the midwife in complicated pregnancies

I do *not* believe that midwives should only be involved in normal pregnancy and birth and that they should not use medical technology. The midwife conducts care of the woman and her family in normal pregnancy and birth on her own responsibility. However, she also has an important role in the care of the family where the woman is experiencing complications. For these women have a right to the midwife's constant presence, the preventative approaches of midwifery, and the emotional support which is an essential component of midwifery care.

Additionally, the skilled midwife is able to use some of our modern-day technology to enhance care. In some situations, the judicious use of technology will enable the mother to proceed to give birth normally and without complications through the reassurance of technological diagnosis. For example, the midwife should be able to order ultrasound examination to assist in accurate dating or assessment of foetal growth. The application of a scalp clip to monitor the heart pattern of a foetus if there have been some indications of distress may enable the mother to give birth slowly with a reassuring heart rate pattern.

In the situation of a woman and her baby experiencing severe complications, the midwife is an important member of the team, working in a different relationship with the parents than the obstetrician. Even with very complex situatons, the midwife, as the advocate for the parents and the child, may maintain emphasis on the human aspects of birth, for even when the birth is surrounded by technology, the child's entry to the world should be marked by respect for the individuality and human rights of each member of the family.

I have become aware of the value of the team approach to care of the woman and her child needing special medical attention, and of the difficulties created when women must be transferred out of midwifery services because they have medical complications. At the time of transfer the woman has often developed a strong relationship with the midwives and, at a time when the occurrence of complications creates great anxiety and grief, she loses their support. This often exaggerates the reactions of anxiety and distrust the woman may experience at such a time.

(3)   ENABLING INFORMED CHOICES

There is nobody who will make more difference to the life of her unborn child than the mother. It is the mother's and the family's daily life and health which have far more effect than any prenatal visits or tests. It makes sense, then, to recognise the parents' central and active role in the care of their child. The midwifery approach should recognise this in giving parents the teaching and counselling they require. If you watch an experienced midwife providing prenatal care, you will see that she is constantly teaching and explaining as she assesses the health of mother and baby. Recognising self-responsibility for care may include such approaches as having the mother weigh herself or testing her own urine.

Remember that the meaning of the word midwife is 'with woman', indicating the closeness of the relationship and the midwife's crucial role in supporting a woman. The midwife is wise advisor, guide and advocate of the family, assisting them to make informed decisions, often nowadays amongst contradictory opinions and confusion within the health care professions. Families also appreciate the friendship of the midwife; she has been called friend and skilled companion. The relationship is a unique one, marked by an intimacy produced by the constancy of care provided.

Midwifery care is also respectful of family integrity: keeping the family intact is one of the major health considerations for the future health of the baby.

(4)   RECOGNITION OF BIRTH AS MORE THAN A MEDICAL EVENT

It is easy in a busy system for physical care to become dominant, and for the other aspects of pregnancy and birth to be forgotten. Concern with the emotional and social as well as physical aspects of care is reflected in the atmosphere of care, in specific words and actions of the midwife, and in the midwifery assessment throughout pregnancy and labour and after the birth.

In the prenatal clinics or visits, the conversation should reflect the understanding the midwife has about the feelings of pregnancy, the ambivalence, the wretchedness of morning sickness, as well as the joy, the anxiety, the disappointment, and the family disruptions of pregnancy. To us the woman is pregnant, to her and her family she is expecting a baby, and we need to find a way in busy, underresourced services, to acknowledge that we understand.

We are beginning to recognise that satisfaction is as important as safety to the successful outcome of pregnancy. But satisfaction is not an adequate word to describe the passion or the fullness of the feelings the parents may experience. The event is physical, but it is also spiritual and sexual, and full of a range of emotions. Not just happiness or joy, but also fear, anxiety, anger and frustration, grief and poignancy surround the experience of pregnancy and birth. In many ways these emotions are those of everyday life, but they are intensified by the significance of the event. For what we see in the faces and actions of the parents as they triumphantly and safely bring their child into the world is much more than satisfaction; it is joy and ecstasy and infinite tenderness.

The midwifery tradition of sensitivity to the spiritual and emotional experience of birth protects these very precious moments, and midwives should be the professionals who restore the right of parents to experience this fullness of birth wherever they choose to deliver.

Perhaps a good motto would be, 'Every birth a home birth.' When, for medical reasons or because it is the family's choice, the parents decide to give birth in hospital, we should ensure that every family is treated in the same way as they would be if they were in their own home. Hospital midwives should enjoy the same autonomy and control as community midwives, and should create an atmosphere which disrupts the family and the processes of pregnancy and birth and postpàrtum as little as possible, while providing the family with as much physical and emotional support as necessary. In this way we may help parents to experience birth in an uninhibited way, knowing a full range of reaction, without being disturbed by the presence of strangers, or by the haste of institutional routines, or by a disapproving atmosphere.

(5) FAMILY-CENTRED CARE

Every family has different needs. In today's world, where every country has a mixed population of different ethnic groups, we are faced with more problems of integration than we have ever known. This is especially true for health care professionals, who must confront problems of communication arising from different languages and different customs, and different ideas about health care and illness.

But it is not just these dramatically different groups of people who require our respect for individual differences. Every person, because of their different backgrounds, different parents and upbringing, and individual personalities, has their own expectations regarding birth and parenting, different dreams, different fears, and hopes.

As with people, all of whom share similar characteristics of personality, physiology and physiognomy, but each of whom is quite unique, each birth shares similar characteristics but is also quite unique.

The development of birth plans may help us in getting to know and acknowledge these differences; the use of continuous care may also help. But also required is a health care service peopled by individuals confident, humane and wise enough to respect individuality, and to protect the care provided by guidelines firm enough to maintain safety, yet flexible enough to provide individual and flexible care.

CONCLUSION

Midwifery care should not be considered inferior medical care, or as a support service for doctors. Instead it should be viewed as a distinct approach to care provided from a unique perspective. Midwifery provides a balance between the family and medical perspectives on birth. To negotiate and balance the different meanings and perspectives of birth within the health care system, it is essential for midwives to have a legitimate and powerful role within the system. Midwifery should be powerful enough to influence both the nature and delivery of services. This, I believe, would greatly enhance maternity care, which ultimately is the crux of the matter, for midwifery is concerned with the safe, loving and skilled care of women, their babies and their families at one of the most important points of life, around the time of birth.

MIDWIVES' ORGANISATIONS

International Confederation of Midwives
10 Barley Mow Passage
Chiswick
London W4 4PH

Australia
Home Birth Access
P.O. Box 66
Broadway
Sydney
NSW 2007

Midwifery Contact Centre (home births)
1a Shoalwater Road
Shoalwater
WA 6169

National Midwives' Association
P.O. Box 1918
Canberra City
ACT 2601

Belgium
Comité de Coordinations des Accoucheuses
Belges d'Expression Française
Les Hauts-Marais
Venelle ND des Champs 70
1300 Louvranges

Brazil
Associacao Brasileira de Obstetrizes
Rue Roberto Dias Lopes 80/302
Rio de Janeiro

Britain
Association of Radical Midwives
62 Greetby Hill
Ormskirk
Lancs L39 2DG

Midwives' Autonomy Action Group
56 Knutsford House
East Mount Street
London E1 1BG

MIDIRS (Midwives' Information and Resource Service)
Westminster Hospital
Dean Ryle Street
London SW1P 2AP

Royal College of Midwives
15 Mansfield Street
London W1M 0BE

Canada
Association of Ontario Midwives
P.O. Box 85, Station C
Toronto
Ontario M6B 3M7

Ontario Task Force on the Implementation of Midwifery
14th Floor, 700 Bay Street
Toronto
Ontario M5G 1Z6

Chile
Colegio de Matronas de Chile
Phillips 15, Depto. L, 6° piso
Santiago

Denmark
Den Almindelige Danske Jordmoderforening
Nørre Voldgade 90
DK-1358 Copenhagen

Finland
Federation of Finnish Midwives
Dagmarisk 12B
0100 Helsinki

France
Association femmes et sages femmes
Permanance Nationale
11–19 rue de la Prevayance
75019 Paris

Greece
Greek Midwives' Association
2 Arist. Pappa., 2 Ampelokipi
Athens 601

Israel
Israel Midwives' Association
P.O. Box 7079
Tel Aviv 61070

Italy
Il Marsupio
Via dei Ginori
40–50129 Firenze

Japan
Japanese Midwives' Association
8–21, I-chome, Fujimi
Chiyoda-ku
Tokyo

Netherlands
Netherlandse Organisatie van Verlofkundigen
Bergmenbosch
Prof. Bromkhorstlan 10
3723 MD Bildhocam

New Zealand
Midwives' Association
24 Ashton Road
Mount Eden
Auckland

USA
American College of Nurse Midwives
1522 K Street NW
Suite 1120
Washington DC 20005

Association of Texas Midwives
Suite 1A– 202
603 West 13th Street
Austin
TE 78701

Bay Area Guild of Midwives
3054 22nd Street
San Francisco
CA 94110

Frontier Nursing Service
Hyden
KY 41749

Illinois Alliance of Midwives
1772 West Estes
Chicago
IL 60626

Maternity Center Association
48 East 92nd Street
New York
NY 10028

Midwives' Alliance of North America
P.O. Box 5337
Cheyenne
WY 82003

Midwives' Association of Washington State
1100 23rd Avenue East
Seattle
WA 98112

New Life Birth Services
1410 West 6th Street
Austin
TE 78703

Oregon Midwifery Council
3839 Pacific Avenue 189
Forest Grove
OR 97116

GLOSSARY

abortion Miscarriage or intentional termination of pregnancy.

ABC Alternative birth centre.

acidosis Condition in which the blood and urine have increased acidity. Also called ketosis (see below).

active birth Labour in which a woman is free to move about and to adopt any positions which she finds comfortable.

active management Method of controlling labour by intervention in order to keep it short.

amniocentesis Puncture of the bag of waters through the mother's abdominal wall and uterus in order to get a sample of amniotic fluid, usually done to test for foetal abnormalities.

analgesia Pain-relieving medication.

antisepsis The prevention of infection.

apgar score System to assess the condition of the baby in the first minutes of life, based on heart rate, breathing, muscle tone, response to stimulation, and skin colour. It is performed at one and five minutes after birth.

artificial rupture of the membranes Amniotomy, the breaking of the bag of waters with small forceps or an amnihook.

asphyxia Suffocation.

augmentation or acceleration of labour Stimulation of the uterus with oxytocin introduced through a vein in the arm.

auscultation Listening to the foetal heart.

bradycardia The slowing of the foetal heart. If it occurs between contracts it may indicate foetal distress.

breech Buttocks-down position of foetus.

cardiography (**cardiotocography**) Graphic representation of relation between the foetal heart rate and uterine contractions.

catheter Tube inserted in a part of the body to introduce or withdraw fluid, or to measure pressure of fluid.

cephalic vertex Head-down position.

cephalo-pelvic disproportion Situation in which the baby's head is too large to descend through the pelvis.

cervix Neck of uterus.

community midwife Midwife who works with GP practice, rather than in team headed by consultant obstetrician.

demerol Pethidine.

direct-entry midwifery Midwifery training which is entirely midwifery-focused, and does not entail first training as a nurse.

diuretic Anything which increases the production of urine.

domiciliary At home. When applied to birth, attendance by a midwife and/or a family doctor, at home.

domino delivery *Dom*iciliary *In O*ut, a British system of care which involves community midwives attending a woman in labour at home, going with her into a consultant unit for the birth, and then returning home six to eight hours after the birth.

eclampsia An acute condition, following pre-eclampsia, in which a pregnant woman or a woman in labour has convulsions.

electronic foetal monitoring The use of electrodes or transducers, either placed over the foetal heart or attached to the foetus, to record the heart rate.

empirical midwife See **lay midwife**.

endorphins Morphine-like substances produced by the body during vigorous exercise, sexual activity, and in any state of high arousal, which reduce sensations of pain.

episiotomy A surgical cut in a woman's perineum to enlarge the birth outlet.

false positive A diagnosis of disease or malfunction which subsequently proves to be incorrect.

foetal distress Hypoxia, or reduced oxygen tension in the body tissues.

foetal growth retardation Slow foetal growth or arrest of growth. Sometimes called intra-uterine growth retardation.

fundus Top of the uterus.

GP unit British maternity unit, or part of a larger unit, in which community midwives and general practitioners are responsible for care.

haemorrhage Excessive bleeding.

hyperemesis Excessive vomiting in pregnancy.

hypertension High blood pressure.

iatrogenic intervention Doctor-produced illness and malfunction.

independent midwife In Britain, a midwife working outside the National Health Service; in North America, a midwife who does not work in a hospital.

induction Starting labour off artificially.

intra-uterine growth retardation A below normal growth rate of the baby inside the uterus.

intravenous infusion Dripping a liquid solution through a catheter into a vein.

intubation Introduction of a tube into the airways.

IV Intravenous infusion.

jaundice Yellow discolouration of skin and eyeballs resulting from breakdown of red blood cells.

ketones Organic compounds resulting from metabolisation of fat in the body.

ketosis An excess of ketones, which can result in acidosis.

lay midwife Midwife who has learnt through practical experience rather than pursuing an established training course.

lithotomy position Delivery position in which woman lies on her back with her legs in the air, bent and wide apart, supported by stirrups.

low-lying placenta Placenta in the lower segment of the uterus.

malpresentation Any presentation of the foetus other than head down.

manual removal of the placenta Introduction of a hand into the uterus to scoop out a retained placenta.

meconium Contents of the foetal bowels, passed in first days of life.

methergin Methylergometrine, drug which stimulates uterine contractions, used to control postpartum bleeding.

multigravida Woman pregnant with second or subsequent baby.

multipara Woman who has had more than one viable baby.

multiple birth Delivery of more than one baby at a time.

NAD Nothing abnormal detected.

neonatal Concerning the newborn baby.

occipito anterior Crown of the foetal head lying towards the mother's front.

occipito posterior Crown of the foetal head lying towards the mother's back, so that the baby is face to pubis.

occiput Crown of the head.

oedema Fluid retention resulting in puffiness.

oxytocin Hormone which stimulates contractions of the uterus.

palpation Examination by touch.

perinatal Around the time of birth.

perineal trauma Injury to the perineum.

perineum Tissues and muscles around and between the vagina and the anus.

pethidine Demerol in the USA, an analgesic drug.

Pinard's stethoscope Traditional trumpet-shaped instrument used to auscultate the foetal heart.

placenta praevia Placenta situated completely or partially over the cervix.

postmature Pregnancy which continues after anticipated date for delivery.

postpartum After the birth.

pre-eclampsia Disease specific to pregnancy in which there is raised blood pressure, albumen in the urine, sudden weight gain and oedema.

premature birth Delivery before 38 weeks from first date of last menstrual period.

presentation The part of the foetus which lies over the cervix.

primagravida Woman pregnant for the first time.

primipara Woman who has given birth to a viable child.

prolapsed cord Emergency in which the umbilical cord has dropped below the level of the presenting part. It results in compression and reduction of the oxygen available to the foetus.

psychoprophylaxis Training of woman for childbirth with strategies for controlling pain, literally by 'mind prevention'. In North America, known as *Lamaze*.

pudendal block Form of anaesthesia in which local anaesthetic is injected around the pudendal nerve.

puerperal fever Acute feverish illness which women suffered historically after childbirth as a result of pelvic infection, the infecting agent often being the doctor's hand.

puerperium Time following birth – six to eight weeks – in which the uterus and other organs return to their pre-pregnancy state.

resuscitation Measures taken to restore to life a baby who is not breathing.

rooming-in Organisation of postpartum care so that mothers can have their babies with them throughout the 24 hours. Often modified to mean during daylight hours only.

rooting reflex Innate tendency of newborn baby to search for the nipple.

scopalamine Hyoscine, analgesic which produces uncontrolled behaviour and delusions.

syntocinon Synthetic oxytocin.

tachycardia Rapid foetal heart rate.

teratogen Substance which when taken by a pregnant woman can cause foetal handicap.

term Due date for delivery.

trial of labour Careful observation of labour in which there is some degree of cephalo-pelvic disproportion and everything is on hand for caesarean section if necessary.

trimester Three-month period.

ultrasonogram Echo-picture.

ultrasound Use of sound waves to bounce off tissues in order to produce an ultrasonogram.

urinary catheter Tube passed into the urethra to draw off urine.

vacuum extraction Method of delivering a baby using a machine that produces suction on the foetal scalp.

CONTRIBUTORS

Lesley Barclay is a midwife and the Education Officer for the Family Planning Association of South Australia.

Hammani Farida is an independent midwife and member of the French Association of Independent Midwives (l'Association Française des Sages-Femmes Liberales). She has practised in Marseilles and is currently working in Garonne, France.

Caroline Flint completed her midwifery training in 1976, and from 1977 to 1980 she worked as a community midwife in Guy's Health District in London. From 1981 to 1986 she was antenatal clinic sister at St George's Hospital, London and then team leader of the 'Know Your Midwife' scheme, a team of four midwives who looked after 250 women each year throughout their pregnancies, labours and the puerperium. In 1986 she began working as an independent home birth midwife and in 1988 joined the Westminster Hospital as a midwifery consultant looking into continuity of care for women and job satisfaction for midwives. Caroline Flint is the author of *Sensitive Midwifery*, and co-author of *The Know Your Midwife Report* and *Community Midwifery: A Practical Guide*. She lives in South London with her husband and three adult children.

Ina May Gaskin founded the Farm Midwifery Center near Summertown, Tennessee in 1971. She and her partners have been responsible for the births of 1,650 babies with low rates of mortality and intervention, such as forceps, vacuum suction and caesarean sections. She is the author of *Spiritual Midwifery* and *Babies, Breastfeeding and Bonding*, and she edits and publishes *The Birth Gazette*, a quarterly magazine. She has produced several video programmes about childbirth and midwifery.

Amanda Hopkinson was born in London where she now lives with her four children. She has been involved in the women's movement since 1968, both in England and in the United States, and has lived and travelled in Central America. She writes on Latin America, women's health and women's photography. Her biography of pioneer photographer *Julia Margaret Cameron* was published in 1986. She has also translated the biography of a fallen guerrilla commander by Salvadorean author Claribel Alegría, *They Won't Take Me Alive*, and is the editor of an anthology of Central American women's poetry.

Susanne Houd trained as a midwife through the direct-entry programme in Copenhagen, and has practised in Denmark and New Zealand. She is currently involved in home birth practice, and is researching post-natal depression, family planning and breastfeeding. She has completed a project on midwives in Europe with Ann Oakley for the World Health Organisation. She is involved in the Danish Midwives' Organisation but works as a privately practising midwife. She has three children.

Astrid Limburg trained as a midwife in Amsterdam and since 1980 has practised there as an independent midwife. She has played an active role in the rediscovery of vertical birth and the promotion of home obstetrics in the Netherlands. In 1983 she designed, with Beatrijs Smulders, the 'Birth-mate', a birthchair to support women in labour. She is Director of the Office of International Affairs and promotes exchange visits between doctors and midwives all over the world. With Beatrijs Smulders, she wrote *Baren* (*Giving Birth*) in 1983.

Frances McConville was born of itinerant parents in Malaysia, and lived variously in Sri Lanka, Canada, Yugoslavia, Ireland and England. After taking a degree in zoology and training as an SRN at Liverpool University, she visited well-woman clinics in California and health centres in Peru and Bolivia. She trained and practised as a midwife at the John Radcliffe Hospital in Oxford until 1984 when she travelled to Bangladesh with Voluntary Service Overseas (VSO). There she established a health programme in the Center for Training and Rehabilitation of Destitute Women in Dhaka and worked with UNICEF as Technical Consultant to the National Traditional Birth Attendant Training Programme. She returned from Bangladesh in 1987 and had her first child that year.

Jutta Mason studied nursing after taking a degree in history and working for two years as a researcher. She worked in large hospitals as well as in an isolated area and, after three years, began to research the history of non-institutional sick care in Canada. The births of her three children focused her interest on the history of non-institutional childbirth and mothering customs, and led her to broaden her enquiry to include the development of medicalised birth and paediatrics in Canada. She is currently writing a book on this subject.

Jo Anne Myers-Ciecko is the Administrator of the Seattle Midwifery School where she teaches a course in the History and Politics of

Midwifery. She has been active in childbirth reform and midwifery politics since the birth of her first child in 1976. She is a board member of the Midwives' Association of Washington State where she edits the state newsletter and served as co-chair of the successful 1987 effort to pass revised midwifery legislation. She is also on the steering committee of the Washington State Healthy Mothers, Healthy Babies Coalition, editor of the *MANA News* (Midwives' Alliance of North America), and serves on the editorial board of the *Northwest Bulletin of Family and Child Health*.

Lesley Page is Director of Midwifery for Oxfordshire, England. She trained as a midwife at the Simpson Memorial Maternity Pavillion in Edinburgh, Scotland and has worked as a midwife in England and in Canada, where she has been active in the movement to legalise midwifery.

Beatrijs Smulders trained as an occupational therapist and as a midwife. She established her own practice as a midwife in 1979 and has since played a leading role in the recent developments of modern obstetrics in the Netherlands. In 1983 she designed, with Astrid Limburg, the 'Birth-mate', a popular birthstool. She has produced numerous films on vertical birth at home and in hospital and has toured the USA to promote active birth and Dutch obstetrics. She is co-author of *Baren* (*Giving Birth*).

Leena Valvanne trained as a nurse, midwife, public health nurse and social worker and she has worked as a nurse and ward sister in Helsinki, as chief medical social worker for the Finnish Population and Family Welfare League, and as a district midwife and supervisor of midwives. Her books include *Maija and Matti's Birth School*, *Your Child is Growing Up*, *The First Moments of Life*, and *Love Without Asking: Memories of a State Midwife*. She is President of the Federation of Finnish Midwives and a member of the Executive Committee of the International Confederation of Midwives, the Council of Europe's study group in Co-ordinated Medical Research and of the World Health Organisation's Perinatal Study Group.

INDEX

Some other Pandora books you might enjoy:

THE TENTATIVE PREGNANCY
Prenatal Diagnosis and the Future of Motherhood

Barbara Katz Rothman

'Anyone who thinks that prenatal diagnosis is liberating for women should read this book.' – Ruth Hubbard, *Harvard University*

More and more women are having children when they are over thirty and amniocentesis, primarily used as a test for Down's Syndrome, is becoming an automatic and routine part of prenatal care.

In this groundbreaking book, Barbara Katz Rothman draws on the experience of over 120 women and a wealth of expert testimony to show how one simple procedure can radically alter the way we think about childbirth and becoming a parent. The results of amniocentesis, and the more recently developed chorion villus sampling, force us to confront agonising dilemmas. What do you do if there is a 'problem' with the foetus? What kind of support can you expect if you decide to raise a handicapped child? How can you come to terms with the termination of a wanted pregnancy?

Passionate, sympathetic and at times heartbreaking, Barbara Katz Rothman's book is a must for anyone thinking of having a child.

'. . . makes women's experience of the technology visible for the first time . . . an immensely intelligent, sensitive and passionate book. No one can read it and remain unmoved.' – Gena Corea

'Wise, sensitive and disturbing – it should be obligatory reading for all health professionals working in this field, and for everyone who wants to understand the increasingly complex face of childbearing in today's world.' – Ann Oakley

£5.95 pbk

THE POLITICS OF BREASTFEEDING

Gabrielle Palmer

This powerful and provocative book shows that breastfeeding is much more than a matter of personal inclination. Women all over the world are still being tricked into feeding their babies artificially and this affects us all: our health, our environment and the global economy.

Gabrielle Palmer asks whether bottlefeeding really does free women to lead more fulfilling lives. She examines social attitudes in a world where a woman who does breastfeed her child risks losing what little income she earns, and alerts us to the commercial reasons behind doctors' recommendations. With an engaging blend of facts, insight and anecdote, Gabrielle Palmer puts infant feeding 'fashions' in their historical and economic contexts. She shows how both poor and rich women suffer the consequences of the male control of a female function. She discusses the ecological effects of the decline in breastfeeding, the nutritional myths and the implications of such issues as AIDS, radioactivity and breast cancer.

The Politics of Breastfeeding challenges our complacency and radically reappraises a subject which is all too often linked only to nursing mothers.

£6.95 pbk

MOTHERHOOD: WHAT IT DOES TO YOUR MIND

Jane Price

'Why didn't anyone tell me it would be like this?'

Having a child is as challenging mentally as it is physically but few of us are prepared for the confusing, often violent, emotions that come with motherhood.

This book is a radically new approach to the psychology of motherhood. Jane Price, herself a mother of two, draws on women's accounts of their feelings at every stage of pregnancy and early motherhood to help us towards a better understanding of those intense emotions which cannot simply be explained away as post-natal depression.

Anger, resentment, guilt and anxiety, jealousy if your baby likes somebody else, fear that you're not 'bonding' properly and an overwhelming sense of inadequacy can make even the sanest woman think she's losing her mind. Jane Price shows how our childhood image of what a mother is – or should be – influences every decision we make: when to have a child in the first place; whether to breastfeed; when, if at all, to return to work. She shows too why women struggle to be at least as good or a great deal better than their own mothers – and why they *think* they fail. Weighing the expectations of parents, partners and friends against our own and never losing sight of the real challenges of being a mother today, Jane Price helps us to accept ourselves – and others – as 'good enough' rather than perfect mothers. She points the way forward to a positive, growing relationship with our children, their father and our own parents.

£4.95 pbk